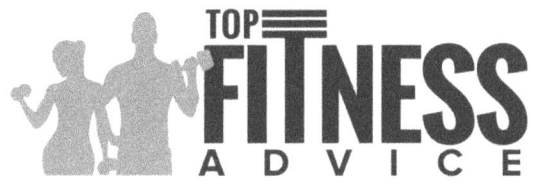

WEIGHT LOSS WORKOUT PLAN

97 Beginner Exercises & Workouts That Target Fat Loss By Burning More Calories In Less Time + 18 Weight Loss Motivation Habits That Help Make You WANT To Work Out Every Day

LINDA WESTWOOD

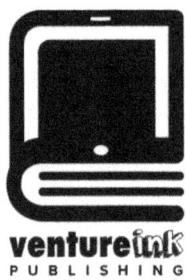
ventureink
PUBLISHING

First published in 2015 by Venture Ink Publishing

Copyright © Top Fitness Advice 2019

All rights reserved.

No part of this book may be reproduced in any form without permission in writing from the author. No part of this publication may be reproduced or transmitted in any form or by any means, mechanic, electronic, photocopying, recording, by any storage or retrieval system, or transmitted by email without the permission in writing from the author and publisher.

Requests to the publisher for permission should be addressed to publishing@ventureink.co

For more information about the contents of this book or questions to the author, please contact Linda Westwood at linda@topfitnessadvice.com

Disclaimer

This book provides wellness management information in an informative and educational manner only, with information that is general in nature and that is not specific to you, the reader. The contents of this book are intended to assist you and other readers in your personal wellness efforts. Consult your physician regarding the applicability of any information provided in this book to you.

Nothing in this book should be construed as personal advice or diagnosis, and must not be used in this manner. The information provided about conditions is general in nature. This information does not cover all possible uses, actions, precautions, side-effects, or interactions of medicines, or medical procedures. The information in this book should not be considered as complete and does not cover all diseases, ailments, physical conditions, or their treatment.

You should consult with your physician before beginning any exercise, weight loss, or health care program. This book should not be used in place of a call or visit to a competent health-care professional. You should consult a health care professional before adopting any of the suggestions in this book or before drawing inferences from it.

Any decision regarding treatment and medication for your condition should be made with the advice and consultation of a qualified health care professional. If you have, or suspect you have, a health-care problem, then you should immediately contact a qualified health care professional for treatment.

No Warranties: The author and publisher don't guarantee or warrant the quality, accuracy, completeness, timeliness, appropriateness or suitability of the information in this book, or of any product or services referenced in this book.

The information in this book is provided on an "as is" basis and the author and publisher make no representations or warranties of any kind with respect to this information. This book may contain inaccuracies, typographical errors, or other errors.

Liability Disclaimer: The publisher, author, and other parties involved in the creation, production, provision of information, or delivery of this book specifically disclaim any responsibility, and shall not be held liable for any damages, claims, injuries, losses, liabilities, costs, or obligations including any direct, indirect, special, incidental, or consequences damages (collectively known as "Damages") whatsoever and howsoever caused, arising out of, or in connection with the use or misuse of the site and the information contained within it, whether such Damages arise in contract, tort, negligence, equity, statute law, or by way of other legal theory.

Table of Contents

Disclaimer	3
Who is this book for?	9
What will this book teach you?	11
Workout Habit #1: Turn Your Commute into A Workout	13
Workout Habit #2: Log Your Workouts	19
Workout Habit #3: Workout with Friends	21
Workout Habit #4: Never Stop Once You Have Momentum	25
Workout Habit #5: Commit For 30 Days	27
Workout Habit #6: Just SHOW UP	29
Workout Habit #7: Schedule Workouts at The Right Times	31
Workout Habit #8: Make It Fun	33
Workout Habit #9: Cross Out Your Calendar	35
Workout Habit #10: Measure & Keep Track	37
Workout Habit #11: Isolate Your Weaknesses	39
Workout Habit #12: Change It Up Regularly	43
Workout Habit #13: Exercise First Thing in The Morning	45
Workout Habit #14: Reward Yourself	47

Workout Habit #15: Higher Intensity Equals Quicker Workouts	49
Workout Habit #16: Don't Put Away Your Gear	51
Workout Habit #17: Invest in Gear	53
Workout Habit #18: Create or Join an Exercise Contest	55
Your Food Plan	57
How You Need to Eat	57
15-Minute Workouts	103
15-Minute Advanced Back Workouts	115
15-Minute Beginner Butt Workouts	131
15-Minute Advanced Butt Workouts	145
15-Minute Beginner Leg Workouts	161
15-Minute Advanced Leg Workouts	177
Proven "Fat-Burn" Exercises	192
Top Tips for Success	267
Conclusion	275
Final Words	279

Would you prefer to listen to my book, rather than read it?

Download the audiobook version for free!

If you go to the special link below and sign up to Audible as a new customer, you can get the audiobook version of my book completely free.

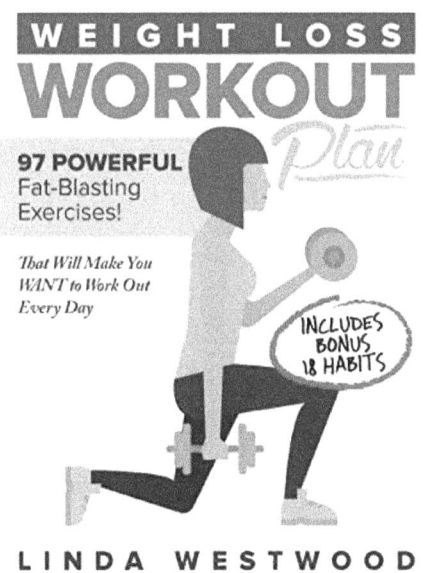

Go here to get your audiobook version for free:

TopFitnessAdvice.com/go/WorkoutPlan

Who is this book for?

Do you feel that your lack of energy stops you from working out?

Are you struggling to stick to healthy habits and lose weight?

Are you one of those people who *know* what to do, but struggle to *actually do* it?

Are you lost when it comes to finding effective workouts that will help you FINALLY lose weight?

Then this book is for you!

I am going to share with you some of the MOST effective workout habits that you can add into your life to lose weight, feel great and have LOTS of energy!

Plus, I am going to share with you over 100 workouts that are PROVEN and EFFECTIVE at burning fat and boosting a person's metabolism!

I have given you a simple action plan at the end of each habit, so you can implement them very easily!

Also, you don't have to be overweight to benefit from these habits.

Yes, they help you lose weight, but they also help you live a healthy life, as well as feel energized throughout your day!

What will this book teach you?

This book is not like others!

It doesn't contain generic advice that we all already know, but actual workout habits that have been identified to INCREASE weight loss, IMPROVE energy levels, and LEAD to a healthier life!

Some of these habits are very simple and you can begin implementing them today, and some are a little more difficult, in that you will need to practice them more!

I will also share with you why each of these habits work and are so effective – along with a simple action plan to help get you started and on your way to lasting success!

And the value of the workout plans themselves alone ARE HUGE because it's going to end the analysis paralysis you are going through in not knowing what you need to do to successfully lose weight FROM TODAY!

Workout Habit #1

Turn Your Commute into A Workout

Many people complain that they do not have enough time in the day in order to get their workout in.

By the time they get up in the morning, get the kids to school, get to work, make dinner, check homework, go to meetings, and tuck the kids into bed, they are way too tired to think about doing a workout.

Finding time to get a workout in when there is so much to do during the day can be difficult. One great place to get in a quick workout is your commute to work.

Instead of driving to work each day, choose to get up and do a workout in order to get there. Some of the ways that you will be able to turn your commute into a workout include:

Running

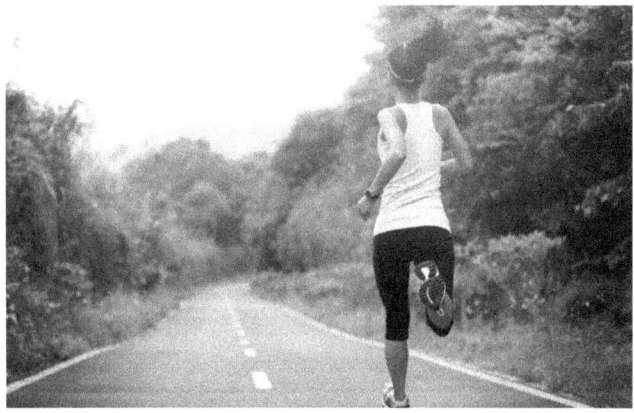

This can get your heart pumping hard and your muscles working. If you live within a few miles of work, you can strap on all of your necessities and make a run of it to work. Do this on the way home as well to get two workouts in and feel so much better about the day.

Cycling

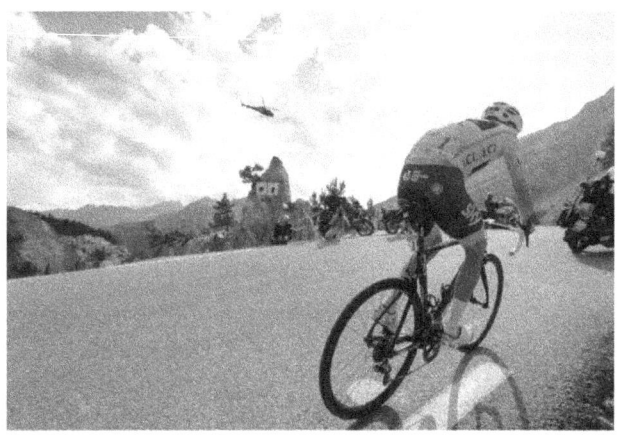

No matter how fast you are going, cycling can be a great workout. Dust off that old bike and give it a ride around the block a few times to get used to it. Cycling can be a good workout that will get you to work fast.

Walking

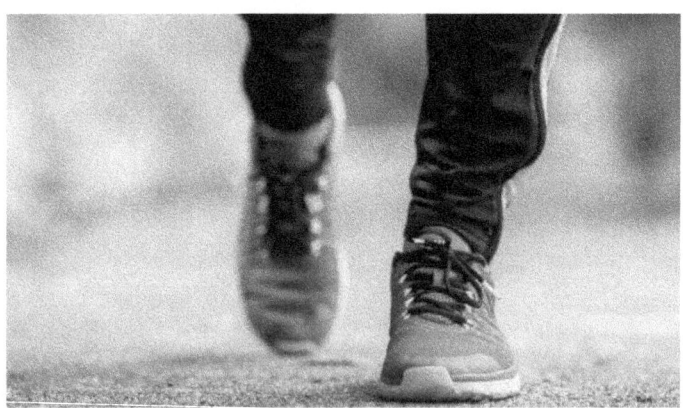

For those who are just beginning their workout routine and are not ready for the things that are more intense, or who live really close to work, walking can be a good option.

Keep up a brisk pace as much as possible to get the heart working to count as the workout.

Driving

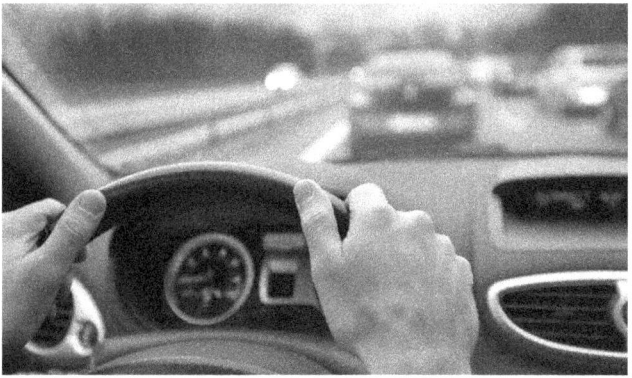

If you do have to drive because you live too far away from work (no one is able to go 30 miles or more to work) you will still be able to get in a good workout.

Park a mile or two away from work and then walk or run to get the rest of the way. This will get you to work on time while still giving you a good workout.

Turning your morning commute is a good way to get up and moving without having to make extra time in the day to add in the workout. Just make sure that you are saving a bit of time to get to work since it will take a bit longer than driving.

You are going to see the results in your health as well as weight loss if you are able to do these exercises, rather than sitting in the car, most days of the week.

Discover Scientifically-Proven "Shortcuts" & "Hacks" to Lose Weight FASTER (With Very Little Effort)

For this month only, you can get Linda's best-selling & most popular book absolutely free – *Weight Loss Secrets You NEED to Know*.

Get Your FREE Copy Here:
TopFitnessAdvice.com/Bonus

Discover scientifically-proven tips to help you lose weight faster and easier than ever before. With this book, readers were able to improve their weight loss results and fitness levels. So, it's highly recommended that you get this book, especially while it's free!

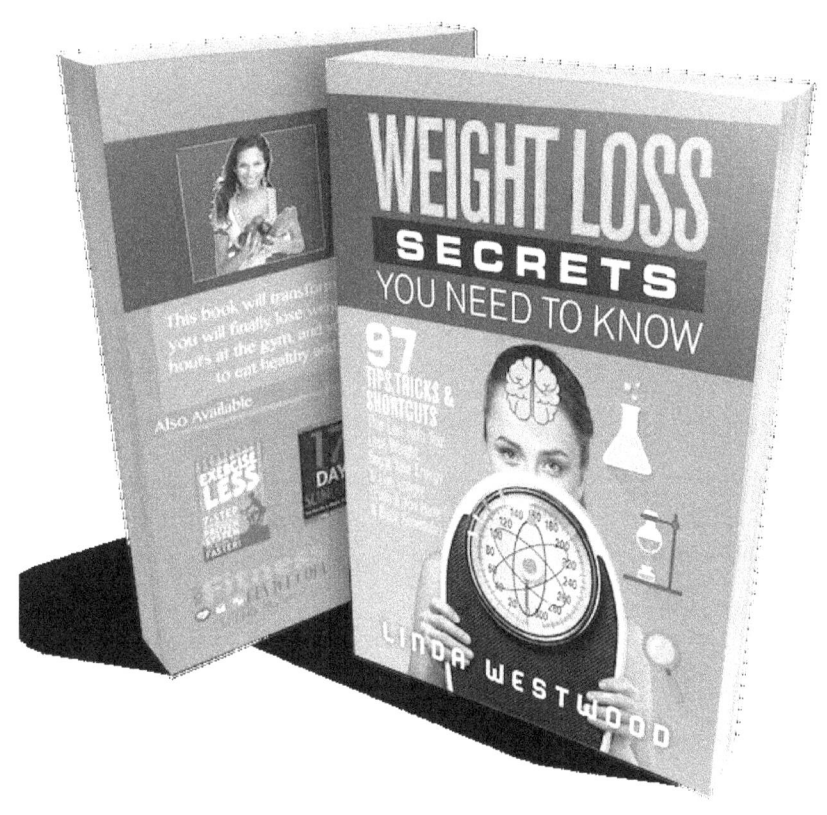

Get Your FREE Copy Here:
TopFitnessAdvice.com/Bonus

Workout Habit #2

Log Your Workouts

Logging your workouts is a good way to ensure that you are actually getting them done each day. It is easy to forget about a workout or two and then by the end of the week, you think that you are doing well but have only done one good workout.

When you log the workouts, you are held accountable for the times you have missed out on and are not doing the best that you can. Now you will know why you are not losing the weight instead of just feeling frustrated that the weight is not coming off like you think it should.

Here are some of the ways that you can track your workouts to makes sure that you are keeping up and giving it your all.

Pedometer

It is recommended that you get at least 10,000 steps into each day for optimal health. Many people, especially those who work at a desk job, find that this number is not even close to what they are actually getting each day.

There are a variety of different pedometers that you can choose from; some are simple and will just calculate the amount of steps that you are taking while others will be more advanced and will include information such as heart rate, calories burned, and amount of time being active.

If you work towards a goal of 10,000 steps each day and try to eat healthy, it is often enough to get your health on track and lose some of the weight that you want.

Fitness Trackers

These are often considered a step up from using the pedometer because they will track more of the things you do than the average pedometer. These will often come with more advanced and will calculate the amount of movement that you do along with your heart rate, and in some cases can tell the difference between the types of movement you are doing, and at the end of the day will tell you a lot of information about your health.

There are several different models including those that go on your wrist, armbands, in your pocket, or on a strap. Be careful with the kind you purchase; some might miscalculate the readings that you get depending on where they are placed. These are a great way to get motivation because you can check any time to see how you are doing and if you need to be doing a little better.

Websites

There are several websites online where you will be able to log your workouts. One of the most popular is myfitnesspal.com. This website allows you to not only calculate the amount of exercise you have done each day, but you can log the foods you ate as well.

Fill out your profile with current information as well as the goals you will like to reach. This website will let you know if you are on track and watches to make sure that you are getting enough exercise and the right nutrition to stay healthy.

Logging the exercise, as well as the food you eat, is a good way to hold yourself accountable to being healthier.

When you can see what you are doing right in front of you it is easier to make adjustments to increase your health or to workout harder.

Workout Habit #3

Workout with Friends

Convincing yourself to get up off the couch and workout can be a hassle. It is much easier to sit there and watch your favorite show with a tub of ice cream than it is to go out in the cold and make it to the gym to work out. Even if you have some equipment in your home, it is difficult to get up and go use it.

One solution that you can try out that will help ensure that you will get up and get that workout done is to do it with friends. Whether you already have a friend who is interested in losing weight as well or you make one at the gym, find someone who is going to motivate you and keep you going no matter what. You will also be able to do the same thing and help them to reach their goals.

Some of the benefits that you will see when you choose to work out with a friend include:

Skipping Less Workouts

When you have someone around to hold you accountable, to keep you motivated, or guilt trip you into showing up rather than abandoning them, you are more likely to get up and go work out. You can meet them at the gym or even go for a nice walk or run together. The activity is not so important as long as you are both doing some form of exercise. When you have someone to meet up with, it is much easier to convince yourself to get up and meet them.

Push each other

Humans are huge competitors so when you are working out with someone else, use this to your advantage. If you see your friend working out hard, try and see if you are able to work out harder. You might not be able to do this all of the time, but you will find that your workouts are much more difficult with someone there.

In addition, if you are having a hard day with working out, your friend will be there to push you, give you encouragement, and ensure that you get the workout done. You should make sure to do the same for them as well.

Try out new things

Doing the same exercises each time you go to the gym will just make them boring and repetitive. You most likely will not keep up with them for the long term and soon your work out goals will be gone.

When you go with a friend, you both might be more willing to try out something new. Your friend might be able to show you a work out they have tried that you will really like or the two of you can try out something that you would not be able to do on your own, such as weight lifting.

Or if there is a new dance class at the gym, maybe your friend will convince you to try it out and you will begin to love this new workout.

Longer workouts

When you go to the gym, it is easy to get going and then say that you are too tired or that you have too much else to do. You might pack it up early and head out the door rather than finish up the work out.

With a friend, you can both set a time for the work out and then you will hold each other to it. No one gets to back out early and both of you will get an amazing workout together.

Recovery together

After a tough work out, it is hard to stay away from those unhealthy foods that are calling your name.

When someone else is going through the issue as well, you can give them a call any time you are feeling weak and discuss the urge. They are most likely going to be able to talk you out of it and keep you on the healthy path.

Having a friend who is willing to work out with you is a great way to ensure that you keep on going at it and reach your health and fitness goals. It is hard to keep up with it on your own and often you will find some excuse or another to not do the workouts you need.

Now with a friend you are held even more accountable and since you do not want to look lazy or disappoint your friend, you are much more likely to get up and get the work done.

Workout Habit #4

Never Stop Once You Have Momentum

Once you get started on an exercise plan and living a healthier life, it can sometimes be difficult to keep it all up. You might spend the first week or two because you are excited about losing the weight and looking your very best.

But after a while, you might find that things get in the way; it becomes easy to take a step away from the healthy workouts and then stop doing them all together. This will then lead to you going back to the old habits you were trying to break.

When you start out on an exercise program, you need to keep at it. It is so good for your life and can help you to get the health and weight loss that you are looking for in your life. But if you stop doing the workouts, you will never see those results. The momentum you get in the beginning is what you will need to carry with you through the rest.

It is hard to convince yourself to keep going as it is but it becomes so much more difficult when you stop for a few days or convince yourself that something else is more important.

Just remember that you have to keep going no matter what. After 30 days, it is going to be much easier because you have made the work outs more of a habit than just something you are forced to do.

If you find that it is hard to get a full work out in all at once each day, you can split them up into smaller increments and still get it all done; a workout that is done during commercials or a bit in the morning and a bit at night will be just as effective as one done all at once.

Gaining momentum can be one of the hardest parts of this whole work out process, but once you get that down, you must keep with it in order to get the best health that you are looking for.

Workout Habit #5

Commit For 30 Days

So, you have decided that it is time to get in shape and improve your overall health, but the idea of working out all of the time and eating healthy frightens you.

How are you supposed to spend a whole lifetime with these healthy habits when your favorite show is calling your name and you really want to eat a second of that dessert?

The secret is that you need to start out slow and steady. Just giving your healthy new lifestyle 30 days makes it more likely that you will turn these choices into habits and you will continue to stick with it for the rest of your life.

30 days and that is it to reach the best health and shape of your life. This is not that long of a time, although it is going to feel like it takes forever when you are first starting.

The first few weeks might seem easy because you are full of energy and excited for the new health and body that you will get, but slowly it is going to sink in that the work is tough and that you are not able to eat everything that comes into your view.

If you can keep going for just a little bit longer, you will reach the goal of 30 days and things will get easier from there on out.

Why the 30 days? Most experts believe that if you are able to do something for 30 days, it will take less effort because it has become a habit. Habits are things you do without necessarily thinking about it because it has become a part of your regular routine.

How nice would it be to not have to think about working out or being healthy because it was just something you got up and did as part of your routine? It is easier than you think if you can just make it through that first 30 days.

It is easy to get the health and wellness that you are looking for in your new workout plan. Whether you are working out every day, five days a week, or going with every other day, you will see results and form a habit if you can commit to just 30 days of your life.

Workout Habit #6

Just SHOW UP

There are going to be days when you are down, are tired from one of the other workouts that you have done, or you just cannot get the motivation that you need in order to get up and go to the gym.

This is the area that a lot of people will fail in; they have all the best intentions, but they are tired or just cannot find the motivation that they need.

Half the battle about getting your work out in is just to show up.

Once you get the shoes on, dressed, and over to the gym you will feel kind of obligated to get up and do something. There are others watching you and it would be kind of silly to put in all of that effort and not do the work out.

So, convincing yourself to do the effort to get to the gym is going to pretty much ensure that you will get in a good work out.

But how do you get yourself to go to the gym? Since this is 90% of the effort that you will need to do for a workout, this is a huge amount of work it seems like it would almost be impossible.

In the first few weeks, you will have the motivation of losing weight and feeling as great as possible. After that time, the motivation is going to go away a bit and it will be a little more difficult to get to the gym.

You will need to find some ways to stay motivated to show up to the gym and get in that great workout. Some ideas that you can try out include:

- Remembering how good it feels to get a workout in.

- Having a friend be there to meet you. It is harder to miss out on a workout if you have someone who is expecting you to be there.

- Have a reward for afterwards. If you make it to the gym, you get to watch your favorite show. If you miss out on the gym, you have to clean the house, car, do the garden or something else. This might motivate you to get out of the house and if not, you are at least still doing some physical activity.

- Pick a time when you are motivated. For some people this is right away in the morning while others do better in the evening. The time does not matter, just pick the one that works the best for your needs and motivation.

No matter what method you choose to use in order to get to the gym, make sure that it is effective.

Just getting out the door and to the gym is the hardest part; once you get that part done, the workout will seem easy in comparison and you will feel great for doing the workout.

Workout Habit #7

Schedule Workouts at The Right Times

At this point, you might be wondering what a good time to do a workout is. Some people think that mornings are the best while others prefer to spend some time in the evening getting in a good sweat before they go to bed. Others think that working out whenever you have the time is the best.

But who is right in all of this? In reality, the time to work out is the one that works the best for you.

If you are a morning person who can get a lot done before heading off to work and school but you are really sluggish in the afternoons and evenings, then working out in the morning is the right time for you.

Others might find that the only time they have free is during nap time for their kids so this is when they will work out and others wait until evening as a way to wind down from the stresses of work and life.

There really is not one ideal time that will work to get in the exercise. The best time is whatever time will work for you.

Some of the things that you should consider when deciding when to work out include:

- ***Are you a morning or evening person***—if you cannot get up well in the morning, evenings might be better for you.

- ***Work***—your work hours are going to determine some of the times you can work out. It is impossible to work out in the morning if you have to be at work by 4 in the morning, but you could fit in an afternoon session when you get off.

- ***Quiet times***—what times of the day work as quiet times in your home? Even if you are able to squeeze in a session during the day, you might be disturbed and have to stop. Find a time when people will leave you alone, where you can put down the phone, and a good work out will get done.

- ***Most motivated***—pick out a time where you are the most motivated to get a workout done. Some people are morning people and this is the best time for them. Others would not be able to function in the morning early enough to do a workout, and so working out at night is a better option.

- ***Nap time***—new mothers and those who stay at home may choose to do this during naptime. They might be up with a baby in the morning and busy or exhausted at night so nap time allows them to get the work out done uninterrupted.

Each person is going to have a different time that works for them to get the exercise they need. Take the time to pick when will work for you and then stick with it as much as possible.

Of course, there will be times when you need to switch it up because something comes up, but keeping the consistency will ensure that you stick with the program for longer.

Regardless of how others do their work outs or when they are able to complete them, you need to do what works for you.

Workout Habit #8

Make It Fun

One of the biggest complaints that people have about exercise is that they find it boring. They feel like they are doing the exact same thing each and every time they go to the gym and it just is not fun.

No one wants to work out or do anything that they do not find fun. But with how important exercise to your life and your health, it is important to include it in each day of your life.

The key here is to make the exercise you are doing fun. You do not want the routine to become too boring or you will quit. This chapter will look at some of the ways you can make exercise more fun and have a great time no matter what.

Group Fitness

There are many gyms who will offer group classes you can join to get your work out. There will be an instructor there who is going to motivate you and others to talk with. You will get an intense work out, make new friends, try something new, and have fun. Take some time to look through your gym to see which classes you might enjoy.

Podcasts and Audio Books

Get a music player and find some podcasts or audio books to download on it. There are hundreds of these available that you can use. The next time that you are about to work out, bring this along and you will be able to keep up with your favorite story while getting some exercise. You can do the same thing with your favorite music.

Chart how it's going

When you chart your progress and the work you are putting in, it becomes easier to have some fun. You can make it a competition to see if you can do better one week after another or if you can at least keep up with the past week.

Try something new

Doing the same thing every day is going to get boring. Try to mix it up every once in a while. For example, if you are used to running on the treadmill each day, take a few nice days and run outside instead. This will prevent the work out from going into a rut and will make it more fun.

Relax

When you are done with the workout, make sure to just relax for at least 5 minutes. Lay down and be completely still and feel how great the work out felt on your whole body.

This is such a great experience that many people miss out on because they are too busy being tired or running around doing other errands during the day. These are just some of the things you can do in order to still have fun while doing something great for your health.

Workout Habit #9

Cross Out Your Calendar

As you are going through getting used to the work outs, you should pull out a calendar and get a big red market.

Each day that you do some form of exercise, whether it is the full one or one that had to be shortened down because you had other things going on, put a big X in the middle of the day.

Each day that you are able to do this there will be an X and you should try to get as many of these X's in a row as possible. The point of doing this is for motivation.

When you see that a lot of days in the week are missing X's, you might feel guilty and realize that you are not doing as well on the working out as you had thought.

On the other hand, if there are a lot of X's on the calendar, you are going to feel pretty good about maintaining your work out.

You will also want to keep the streak going and will work out harder to keep it going. It is a great motivational tool to keep things going in the right direction.

Workout Habit #10

Measure & Keep Track

While you are working out, you need to make sure that you are properly measuring and keeping track of the progress you are making. There really is no reason for you to be doing all of this if you do not have some measuring stick for how well it is going or if you need to try harder.

The great thing about this is that you will be able to pick how you would like to measure it. You could do measurements of the body, such as with your hips, waist, thighs, and arms, or you can go by weight. You can even just go by the way that you feel or if a health condition is being improved.

This chapter is going to spend some time looking through the different ways that you can measure and keep track of the work outs you are doing to ensure that you are getting the most out of each one.

Weight

The most common way people will choose to monitor their progress is with the amount of weight that they are losing. They want to get their weight down to a certain number so that they look better and have better health.

When measuring by weight, you need to remember to weigh yourself at the same time every session. You are going to weight different amounts throughout the day depending on the amount of food you eat and other factors. If you weigh in the morning before breakfast the first time, it is best to keep with this each time you do it.

It is usually best to weigh yourself once a week to keep track and to see any results.

Body measurements

This is the one that is the most commonly recommended. Sometimes the scale will not show the numbers that you want and it might even go up a bit even when you are working really hard to lose the weight.

This can be discouraging. It is not that you are necessarily gaining back the weight or doing a poor job, it is more the fact that you are gaining muscle; muscle weighs more than fat.

A good way to still see the progress you are making is to take body measurements. Once a week, measure the stomach, hips, thighs, and arms to see if they are getting smaller. Even though the scale might not agree, these numbers will still be going down when you do a good work out.

Improvement of health

There are many different health conditions that can be improved when you start working out. You can measure your success based on how well you are able to manage the health conditions you already have.

Talk with your doctor and go in for your regular checkups to ensure you are taking the proper care of your body.

I hope that you are enjoying this book so far, and if you could spare 30 seconds, I would greatly appreciate you leaving a review on Amazon.com.

Workout Habit #11

Isolate Your Weaknesses

When it comes to improving your health, you will find that there are a million little things that you can change about yourself.

You might find that you do not drink enough water, your diet is not healthy, you eat too many snacks, or you do not work out enough.

While it is noble to want to attack all of these things at once and get back into good health overnight, this is a little over ambitious and often you will find that you are failing.

A better approach is to take things one at a time. Find out what a few of your weaknesses are and then attack them slowly.

Maybe start with getting rid of the soda first and after you are used to that, you can add in a little more exercise and so on. Doing it one thing at a time makes the task more manageable and you will be more likely to do it.

The change in your routine only has to happen slowly. Doing a few small changes is often enough to get it all started. Some of the small changes you can do include:

Go for a walk before supper

This is something simple that you can do with your family that gets you up and moving. The walk does not have to be long or that vigorous, just get up and move a little. You can do this either before or after supper and head to the park to play for a bit.

Keep a bottle of water

Drinking plenty of water is the best way to keep your health up, but it is easy to forget to drink enough. Keeping that water handy makes it easy to grab a drink when you need it and seeing the bottle there keeps it at the front of your mind.

Hide the remote

It is easy to get lost in the TV every night and pass hours watching it. This is not going to get you the exercise that you need and is often going to make you eat more. Hide the remote and get up and do something with your family.

Take a lunch to work

This will help you to avoid going out to eat every day and packing on the calories; something that is easy to do when you are busy at work and hungry.

Walk to the store

Instead of driving to the store that is five blocks away to pick up a gallon of milk, why not walk to get there. This is some great exercise that will get you up and moving in no time and this simple errand will add an extra mile in your day.

Cut out the soda

Many people will consume a lot of soda in their day. This can really add up the calories and can make it hard to lose the weight that you want. Cut this out and be amazed how easily the weight comes off.

Cut the sweets

Many of the sweets you eat will have more calories than you would have thought. Make sure to limit those to just once or twice a week for the best results.

Start slow

You do not have to run a marathon every day for your work out. Do just a few simple things, like the ideas listed above, and you will be amazed at the results.

These are just some of the of the things you can consider doing, one at a time, to improve your health and make sure that you are looking and feeling your very best.

Workout Habit #12

Change It Up Regularly

When you find something you enjoy doing for a work out, it is easy to get into a routine of just doing this each and every day.

While it is great that you enjoy it, you are eventually going to stop seeing the results. This is because your body is going to start getting used to the routine and it will become so efficient at doing all of this that the results will not be seen.

Changing up the routine you do can ensure that your body is getting a fantastic work out all of the time.

Why change it up

As mentioned, when you do the same workout all of the time, your body is going to stagnate at one place because it is so used to doing it. It is nice to have a workout that seems to be doing wonders for your body, but after a few months, that is going to go away.

When you change up the routine, you are making sure that you never get bored, you continue to see results, and you are motivated to keep going.

How often

This will often depend on what you are looking for. Some people will suggest that you do a different activity each day. This might be a lot of work to find several work outs that you like all of the time. You will still be able to see some results if you change it up once or twice a month.

Just remember, you can go back to some of the old exercises that you did in order to enjoy them again once you have been off them for a while.

How to change

You might have to be a little bit creative in order to change up the routine. You will want to find some fun activities that you enjoy doing and add those into the routine. Trying out something new can be a lot of fun as well.

Workout Habit #13

Exercise First Thing in The Morning

It is possible to work out at any time of the day that fits into your schedule. It is much better to get a work out in to the day rather than miss it because you were not able to do it at a certain time.

On the other hand, if you happen to have a choice in the time you work out, many experts agree that you should consider working out right away in the morning.

Some of the reasons why you should work out in the morning include:

1. ***Better results for the long term***—those who work out in the morning seem to be more consistent compared to those who do it later on in the day.

2. ***Fewer conflicts in the schedule***—as the day goes on, more things are going to get into your way and soon you may find there is no time for working out. If you do a work out right away in the morning, there has not been enough time for things to get in the way.

3. ***Higher productivity***—after a morning workout, you will be able to get more done. You will feel more awake and will be able to tackle the whole day because you have more energy.

4. ***Better metabolism***—you are going to continue to burn more calories even after you are done with the work out. Use this during the day while you are eating rather than

having it go while you are asleep and everything is slowed down anyway.

5. **Better sleep** – those who get up earlier to work out will have better sleep. This is mostly due to the fact that exercise can wake you up with the endorphins released; this means that exercising at night can actually wake you up and keep you awake.

6. **Better diet**—when you do a work out in the morning, you are going to be more conscious of the foods you are eating in the day. You do not want to sabotage the hard work you did so you will make smarter choices in your diet.

Workout Habit #14

Reward Yourself

Working out is tough to do. You have to convince yourself to get up and move, even though you are tired and want to be doing something else with your day. But it is so good for the heart and your overall health that you have to get it in at least most days of the week.

This does not mean that working out has to be a punishment. In fact, you should make sure to reward yourself for all of the hard work you have put into your workouts.

This gives you even more motivation to keep on going even when it is getting tough or you would rather just stay in bed just a little bit longer.

There are several ways you can measure your accomplishments in order to get a reward. You can say that if you work out every day for two weeks you get a reward or once you lose the first five pounds.

Have several reward systems in place so that you have even more to look forward to even when the going is starting to get hard. This is going to be another motivational tool that you can use in order to feel great and still get that work out in no matter how hard it might get.

You will be able to pick the kind of reward you would like to give to yourself. Pick one that is going to actually be appealing to you so that you work harder.

Choosing a big prize that you do not actually care about really is not going to be a good motivational tool when you hear that screeching alarm clock in the morning. Some ideas you can use for your reward include:

Clothes

After you lose so much weight, promise to go out and pick some new and nice clothes that will fit your new body and make you feel amazing.

See a movie

Go out for a girls' night or with your special someone to see a move as long as you got enough work outs in for the month.

Spa day

All that working out is exhausting. Why not treat yourself to a nice day at the spa. Go on your own to enjoy some quiet time or take a few friends to have some fun.

Do not use food

Using food as an incentive is a bad idea, especially if you are trying to use weight. You can have a treat on occasion, but keep it to a minimum and do not use it as an incentive when working out.

Workout Habit #15

Higher Intensity Equals Quicker Workouts

Long workouts are boring and take up a lot of your time. Not everyone has hours each day to go to the gym and get the work out and burn the calories they need.

Instead of wasting all of that time at the gym each day, why not consider getting into a higher intensity work out. These are great because they allow you to get the same kind of work out, burn the same if not more calories, but you can spend a lot less time at the gym.

Some of the benefits that you will see with doing these kinds of workouts include:

1. *Efficient*—the first thing that you will notice with these kinds of exercises is that they are more efficient. Instead of spending an hour at the gym walking 3 miles, you can spend a little over half an hour jogging 4 miles. You get more in but it is all done in less time.

2. *Burn more fat*—the harder you work out, the more fat you will be able to burn. The fat is what is going around your hips and thighs and something you will really want to get rid of if you are trying to lose weight. It is also healthier for your overall health.

3. *Healthier heart*—intense exercise is great at making your heart pump faster and growing this

important muscle. Clearing out the fat in your body can also help with lowering the risk of stroke and other heart diseases.

4. ***Lose the weight not the muscle***—you are burning a lot of calories when you are doing high intensity workouts, but the muscle is still going to be there. This allows you to keep a lean frame while still losing weight.

5. ***Higher metabolism***—high intensity work outs can increase your metabolism even more than normal work outs. This means that long after you are done working out, you will be able to continue to burn calories and lose more weight.

Workout Habit #16

Don't Put Away Your Gear

Many people will end up placing their gear away when they are done working out. This allows it to be out of the way, but is not very conducive to working out the next day. When the gear is put away, it is easier to forget about it or think that it is too difficult to go get it out.

On the other hand, if you leave the gear out so that you can see it or it is at least in the way, you are more likely to get up and go to the gym to use it.

Make sure that you are putting the gear in a place where it is not right in the way of everyone, but you are sure to see it and be reminded to go to the gym.

Leave it by the side of your bed so it is something that you will see first thing in the morning. Or you can place it right by the front door if you have a sunroom to put it in.

The area is not as important as making sure that you are able to see it as a reminder to go work out.

Workout Habit #17

Invest in Gear

If you are really serious about getting into shape and starting a new workout routine, it is best if you spend a little bit of money and invest in the gear that you will need in order to get it done.

This does not have to be a huge investment but it is still good to have some quality gear. This is going to make you look good, help you to stay motivated to get the workout done, and can be great at keeping you safe.

This chapter is going to look at some of the gear you should consider investing in to get the most out of your workouts.

Workout clothes

These do not have to be really expensive or designer in order to work, but having a designated pair of clothes that you wear when it is time to work out can help a lot.

This is a good way to put your mind in the mode that it is time to work out; wearing your street clothes might make it more difficult to be focused.

A good pair of sweats or running shorts and a t-shirt will work out just as well as any expensive brand, just make sure that you save this outfit just for your exercise.

Shoes

It is time to invest in a good pair of running shoes. Even if you plan to do a lot of biking or weight lifting, you still need a good pair of shoes in order to stay safe and ensure that you are not pulling or twisting anything. Find a pair of shoes that has good support and that you can wear comfortably while doing some strenuous activity.

Stop Watch

Use this to measure the actual amount of time that you are spending working out. It is easy to stop working out in order to answer a text message or to do something else. You might be surprised at how little you are getting done.

Use the stopwatch to make sure that you are actually getting the workout that you want done.

Music player

Music is a great way to get in a work out and keep motivated. Pick your favorite playlist with a lot of high speed and loud music to keep you on the right pace. Many people like to listen to music to make sure that they are keeping pace or to keep them entertained while working out.

Pedometer or tracker

This is a great option to have because it can keep track of all the activity that you are doing during throughout the day. You can get a variety of trackers depending on the needs that you have with using it.

Pick one that works well for you, whether you just want to track your steps each day or you are interested in also calculating heart rate, activity, and calories burned.

Workout Habit #18

Create or Join an Exercise Contest

Another way that you will be able to get the work outs that you want and lose the weight is to either create or join an exercise contest.

These bring out the natural competition that most people have and makes it more likely that you will be able to stick with the plan. Everyone wants to do better than someone else and these competitions will allow you to do just that.

If you are creating your own competition, it is probably best to just stick with doing it with friends and family.

Find some others you know who are working to exercise more or to lose weight and see if they are interested in competing against each other to see who is able to do the best with it over a certain amount of time.

You can agree on the amount of time before you start, how you will calculate the results (who has lost the most weight, who lost the biggest percentage of weight, or who worked out the most), as well as a prize for the winner.

There are also many towns who will have yearly competitions. You sometimes have to be a part of their gym, but often they will open the competition to anyone who wants to join in and try to get healthier.

You should make sure to read through all of the rules that are given to figure out if this is the right step for you or if something else would work out a little better.

Most of these competitions will have times when you will need to report your results and there will be a prize that is available.

When it comes to a premade competition, the prize will be picked out ahead of time and you will know what you are working out for the whole time.

This allows you to have some motivation of being the best and getting that prize. If you are doing this with your friends and family, pick out a prize between you all before you get started.

You could get a gift card to a spa and offer it to the winner or something along those lines. Using competition to motivate yourself to work out and be healthier is a great option.

Humans like to compete and you will find that your competitive nature will come out like crazy when the competition comes up. You will find it is easier to get off the couch and go to the gym or eat healthier because you want to see those results and you want to do better than everyone else.

Use this to your advantage and you will slowly start to build the habits that you need in order to keep doing this for the long term.

Your Food Plan

How You Need to Eat

Before you start any workout plan, it's important to get your diet under control.

Food is not just calories you put into your body to keep going. It's full of vitamins, minerals, fatty acids, and macronutrients that your body depends on to repair itself and to operate at peak efficiency.

If you don't eat a healthy and balanced diet, you will not only be gaining weight (in pure fat), you'll also be preventing your body from getting the most out of the workouts you do.

Your muscles depend on certain specific nutrients in order to grow and become stronger.
If you aren't getting those nutrients from your diet, you will literally be starving your muscles and no amount of exercise is going to change that.

Without diet, you'll quickly hit a plateau in your workout and be unable to burn more fat or gain more muscle. You'll be stuck halfway to your goal and find that making any more progress is an unwinnable uphill battle.

If you eat mostly processed foods and snack on junk food, you might feel full but your body is still starving. These are empty calories that pack on weight without adding any nutritional value.

In the next section, you'll get a brief introduction into nutrition. We'll talk about which nutrients are important for which parts of the body and some natural food sources where you can find them.

We'll also take a closer look at how your body burns fat and builds muscle and what it needs in order to do those things effectively.

After you've finished reading through this brief crash course in nutrition, you'll get 4 sample meal plans which you can copy directly or modify to your own needs.

Each meal plan covers an entire week of breakfasts, lunches, dinners, and even snacks so that eating healthy doesn't have to be a constant source of worry for you.

With these meal plans, you can plan your grocery shopping right to avoid having to stress about what to buy and whether or not you've got all your nutritional bases covered.

Finally, you'll get 10 surprisingly easy and delicious recipes to get you inspired to break out of your processed junk food rut and explore the full flavor potential of healthy food.

Eating healthy doesn't have to be bland and boring. In fact, it can be even more exciting than your favorite junk foods.

Altogether, this chapter will help you make a complete and smooth transition to a healthy diet by taking all the guesswork out of it. Think of it is an all-in-one starter kit to help you eat healthy. Once you get started, maintaining the diet will only get easier and easier as your tastes change and you start to appreciate the rich flavors of nutritious food.

A Basic Guide to Nutrition for Fat Loss and Body Sculpting

You probably already know all too well that a poor diet leads to weight gain. But there are a lot of myths and misinformation out there about exactly how your weight and diet are connected. Most people believe that eating fat is what makes you fat. But this is not necessarily true.

The simple fact is that you gain weight when you eat *more* calories than you burn. It doesn't matter whether those calories come from fat, protein, carbohydrates, or anything else.

If you eat 3,000 calories of anything and then only burn off 1,800 calories, the remaining 1,200 calories will get stored as fat. That's how weight gain happens.

Now, that doesn't mean you have to spend the rest of your life counting every single calorie that goes in your mouth. That is stressful, tedious, and not really necessary.

If you want to eat *less* calories than you burn so that you lose weight or the *same* amount of calories that you burn so that you maintain your weight, all you have to do is watch where those calories are coming from.

When you eat a diet full of empty calories (high caloric foods with low nutrition value), you are going to eat more calories. This is because the number of calories your meal contains has nothing to do with how full you will feel in the end.

One small bag of potato chips contains an average of 1,200 calories. That's more than half of an average 2,000 calorie diet! But after eating that small, snack-sized bag of chips, you definitely don't feel like you ate half a day's worth of food.

On the other hand, the recipe for BBQ baked beans with sweet potatoes that you'll find below contains just 530 calories per serving and is guaranteed to make you feel completely full after you finish eating.

That recipe (along with all the other recipes) is not specially crafted to be low in calories. You'll notice that all the recipes tend to call for full fat, full calorie versions of the ingredients.

The reason that 530 calories of baked beans will leave you feeling fuller than 2,000 calories of potato chips is that the baked beans are packed with protein, fiber, and unsaturated fats (the good fats).

On top of that, they're loaded with the vitamins and minerals your body needs. Potato chips, on the other hand, have no nutritional value and are full of saturated and Trans fats (the bad fats).

So, **rule #1 of healthy eating for weight loss: count nutrients, not calories.**

If your meal is full of the nutrients your body needs, it will feel satisfied for a lot longer, meaning you'll eat less total calories in the long run. So, don't bother with low fat or "diet" versions of food. There's no reason to sacrifice flavor just to lose weight.

In fact, you'll lose *more* weight by eating the real versions of food than their "diet" versions because real food leaves you feeling more satisfied.

The right diet can also help rev up your metabolism so that you burn more calories, even while resting. Fiber for your digestive system is like oil for your car's motor.

Without it, everything gets blocked up and can't move through. Making sure you get enough fiber in your diet will help make sure that your digestive system doesn't get backed up which means that it can process food more efficiently.

The average American diet does not contain even half of the fiber you should be eating each day. You need about 30 grams of fiber every day on average—more if you eat a high protein diet (more than 70 grams of protein per day).

So, **rule #2 of healthy eating for weight loss: eat at least 30 grams of fiber per day.**

Water is also essential for your metabolism—and for your entire body, actually. You should be drinking *2 liters* of water per day. This is the amount your body needs to stay hydrated.

Making sure that you are hydrated will help improve your blood circulation, improve digestion, boost metabolism, keep you energized, and reduce the frequency of headaches.

The overwhelming majority of Americans are chronically dehydrated. Dehydration leads to slowed metabolism, slowed blood circulation (which means less oxygen to the muscles), fatigue, headaches, and other, even more serious health problems.

This brings us to **rule #3 of healthy eating for weight loss: drink 2 liters of water every single day!**

Drinking 1 or 2 glasses of water right when you wake up is a great way to kick start your metabolism. One little known fact about weight loss is the importance of muscle mass. The majority of people focus only on burning fat and don't really pay any attention to gaining muscle.

This is because their focus is on making the number on the scale go down, not on shrinking their waistline. But muscle weighs more than fat. That means the precise number of pounds doesn't matter as much. There will come a point in your workout where your weight stops going down (or even starts going up) even though you aren't actually getting bigger.

Embrace this. The more muscle you have, the better. That doesn't mean you need to become a bulky bodybuilder. It just means you need to incorporate strength training into your workout so that you are gaining muscle at the same time as you are burning fat.

The more muscle you gain, the more quickly you burn fat. This is because muscle burns more calories, even when your body is at rest. So, the more muscle you have, the more fat you will burn. So rather than focusing on burning fat, focus on building muscle. By doing that, the fat will burn off naturally.

One way to do this is to set a goal for your waistline rather than your weight. You can still step on the scale to check your progress but taking regularly measures of your waistline will give you a better idea of the progress you are making.

That brings us to **rule #4 of healthy eating for weight loss: eat a high protein diet.**

Your muscles need protein in order to grow and get strong. The average person—which means someone who doesn't really exercise—needs 50 to 60 grams of protein per day.

Once you start incorporating the workout routines from this book, however, you will no longer count as the "average person." You need more protein to make sure your muscles can keep up with your new workout schedule.

You should be eating ½ a gram to 1 gram of protein per pound of body weight every day in order to make sure your muscles have enough nutrients to rebuild and to stay strong. If you weigh, say, 150 pounds, you would need to eat between 75 and 150 grams of protein per day.

Remember, if you increase your protein, you should increase your fiber. Rather than 30 grams of fiber per day, try to get between 40-50 grams in order to make sure your digestive system can handle the increased protein (which is the most difficult nutrient to digest).

In essence, what you need to achieve with your diet is balance. You want the right proportions of protein, carbohydrates (including fiber), and unsaturated fats. The standard recommended proportions are 30% protein, 50% carbohydrates, and 20% unsaturated fats.

That means, whatever your total number of calories ends up being, 30% of them should come from protein, 50% from carbohydrates, and 20% should come from fats.

Again, you don't need to count calories, just count nutrients. By making sure you get enough of those 3 macronutrients from healthy, whole foods rather than processed junk, you'll be able to easily insure that you are giving your body everything it needs.

This brings us to our final rule, **rule #5 of healthy eating for weight loss: balance and variety are the spice of life.**

In order to make sure you get all your vitamins and minerals in addition to the macronutrients (protein, fiber, unsaturated fats), make sure your diet is varied.

Don't just eat beef to get your protein. Include fish, chicken, beans, nuts, and seeds as well.

Don't just eat cheese or dairy to get your healthy fats, eat vegetable oils (especially olive, almond, coconut, or flaxseed oil) and other fatty or oily foods (like avocados, fish, nuts, or eggs).

You don't need to tediously work through the list of vitamins and minerals that each ingredient on your plat contains. Just make sure you eat a wide variety of whole, unprocessed foods with a focus on achieving that macronutrient balance you read about earlier (30/50/20).

Now that we've taken a quick look at the 5 key rules of healthy eating for weight loss, let's start looking at some of the myths of healthy eating and why they are false. The point of this section is to help you realize that a healthy diet is far from bland and boring.

A lot of healthy foods that also taste delicious have gotten an undeserved bad reputation due largely to outdated science and a poor understanding of nutrition and health.

Here is the good news about healthy dieting:

Myth #1: Diets need to be low in fat and high in carbohydrates

If you stumble across a diet that tells you to cut out fat and boost carbohydrates, steer clear. As you read earlier, eating fat does not make you fat.

Any diet that tells you to cut out or dramatically decrease the amount of one category of food should be avoided. In fact, "diets" should be avoided. Instead, aim for a healthy *balance* of whole, unprocessed foods.

More importantly, not all carbohydrates are created equal. Simple carbohydrates (like refined flour, starches, and sugar) lead to sharp spikes and drops in your blood sugar levels which give you sudden bursts of energy followed by sudden fatigue and cravings for food.

This can lead to you eating more calories in the long run (which will cause *more* weight gain). That is not to say that you should cut out carbohydrates. Just focus on complex carbohydrates.

Typically, those are foods high in fiber. The more carbohydrates that come from fiber (rather than sugar), the healthier it is for you. So, don't cut fat in favor of carbohydrates and make sure that the carbohydrates you eat are primarily complex carbohydrates (high fiber, whole grains, whole foods, and so on).

Myth #2: Eggs are bad for you

It seems almost like common knowledge now: eggs are high in cholesterol, therefore, don't eat eggs. But this is the furthest thing from the truth. Yes, eggs are high in cholesterol but that cholesterol is HDL—the good kind. Your body actually needs HDL cholesterol in order to function.

This is because HDL cholesterol acts as a sort of LDL (bad) cholesterol hunter. It cleans the LDL cholesterol—which is what clogs your arteries and veins—and transports it to your liver where it can be broken down and removed.

That means that eggs actually *lower* your bad cholesterol. So, you no longer have to punish yourself by avoiding eggs. Eat eggs every day as often as you want!

There also loaded with protein and other essential nutrients. They are one of the most complete foods you could eat.

Myth #3: Coffee is bad for you

This myth is partially true. If you drink a lot of coffee (more than 2 cups per day), then you are putting yourself at risk. Too much coffee does cause increased heart rate and higher blood pressure. It can also cause problems with sleeping if you drink it too close to bed time. That's because it's a stimulant.

But 1 or 2 cups of coffee per day are not going to cause any of these negative health problems because it's not strong enough in that amount. Contrary to causing problems, 1 or 2 cups per day is actually *beneficial* to your health.

A cup of coffee in the morning wakes up your metabolism and helps your digestion which leads to increased weight loss (and explains the tendency to need to use the bathroom after a morning java boost).

Coffee is also naturally free of calories so if you skip the cream and sugar, it's the perfect 0 calorie way to get an energy boost. It also contains important antioxidants which help prevent cancer.

If that wasn't enough, some recent studies are also starting to show that it might actually help prevent type 2 diabetes! So, drink up and enjoy (but don't go overboard).

If you have a habit of going heavy on the cream and sugar, start weaning yourself off those additives by gradually decreasing the amount you put in (especially the sugar). Learn to appreciate the bold cancer-fighting flavor of black coffee!

Myth #4: High protein diets are always unsafe

If you exercise regularly (especially if you are strength training), the bottom line is you *need* more protein. Protein is absolutely essential for muscle growth so it's kind of strange that it gets such a bad reputation.

It is claimed that too much protein leads to kidney failure. If you already have preexisting kidney problems, then yes, you should eat less protein. But otherwise, there are no studies which show protein *causing* kidney problems.

One issue with high protein diets is that they often tell you to cut carbohydrates in favor of more protein. As you read earlier, *any* diet that tells you to cut out a food group should be avoided.

In the case of high protein diets, you also need to increase your complex carbohydrates.

Eating more protein means you also need to eat more fiber so that your digestive system can handle it. Again, what it comes down to is balance. There is no amount of protein that is unhealthy just as there is no amount of fiber that is unhealthy.

The health risks start when the *balance* of these macronutrients is off. Too much protein without enough fiber will lead to constipation and overload of difficult to process food without the nutrients it needs to actually process them.

Myth #5: Low fat foods are good for you

This is one of the most rampant and dangerous health myths out there. Foods that are naturally low in fat are safe and often even healthy, sure. But foods that *should* be high in fat but have had that fat removed are usually horribly bad for you and cause even more weight gain to boot.

This is because when manufacturers remove fat from a food that should have fat in it, it tends to taste horrible or, at best, overwhelmingly bland.

In order to make up for that lack of flavor, manufacturers usually just pour in loads of sugar. Sugar is extremely unhealthy. Not only does it lead to weight gain, it can cause diabetes, headaches, and fatigue (from the sugar crashes).

Always, *always* choose the full fat version of food. By the same logic, always choose the "no sugar added" versions of food. Processed foods hide unimaginable quantities of sugar.

In most cases, there is even sugar added to the vegetables of a TV dinner which totally counteracts the nutrition value of those vegetables. Just avoid processed foods—which includes foods that have reduced fat or market themselves as "diet" foods. You want whole foods like produce, meat, eggs, dairy, nuts, and seeds. You want foods that don't have a huge list of ingredients (especially when those ingredients are things you can't pronounce or can't immediately identify).

Myth #6: Avocados are bad for you

Some people think that the high fat content of avocados makes them bad for you—ditto for nuts and seeds. In fact, all of these are extremely good for you.

First of all, the fat content is almost exclusively unsaturated fat (the healthy fats). Not only does healthy fat contribute to weight loss (by boosting the metabolism), it also does wonders for your skin. Your skin actually needs fat in order to stay moisturized, reduce wrinkles, and avoid cellulite.

If you were to cut out all fat from your diet, your skin would soon become dry, scaly, wrinkled, and just generally unappealing. No amount of moisturizers and lotions would help because your skin needs to get fat from your diet (not from lotion).

The same way your skin would become dry and scaly, your hair would also start to get dull and brittle. Healthy fats are what give your hair natural shine and body.

So, while you need to cut out Trans fats (which are artificial and extremely bad) and moderate your saturated fats (which are safe in controlled amounts), you should be boosting your unsaturated fats.

Remember to maintain the right balance (30/50/20) with protein and carbohydrates, though. So, eat avocados, nuts, and seeds to your heart's content! They are also high in vitamin E and other antioxidants which also keep your skin smooth and healthy (and prevent cancer at the same time).

Plus, recent studies have shown that avocados improve your body's ability to absorb other nutrients. That means adding avocado to your meal will help improve the amount of nutrients you absorb from all the other foods on your plate, too!

Myth #7: Chocolate is a junk food

Those of you with a serious sweet tooth will be overjoyed to learn that not only is chocolate *not* bad for you, it is actually extremely healthy!

Of course, when we talk about chocolate, we mean the actual chocolate content, not the sugar and cream that are usually added to candy bars.

But a rich, flavorful bar of dark chocolate (at least 70% cacao) is full of cancer-fighting antioxidants. Plus, it contains compounds that naturally boost your mood. A few ounces of chocolate a day keeps the doctor (and the blues) away!

As with coffee, though, you don't want to overdo it and you want to cut the amount of added sugar as much as possible. Try melting down your daily dose of dark chocolate and dipping strawberries or other yummy (and healthy) fruits to make an extra special, extra healthy treat!

Myth #8: Alcohol should be avoided entirely

Let's start by clarifying that this book is absolutely *not* advocating a bottle of vodka a day or even a night of binge drinking. Too much alcohol is definitely a bad thing and can lead to extremely serious problems as well as extremely embarrassing moments.

The myth this book is talking about is the myth that you should not drink any alcohol at all, ever. But, just like coffee or chocolate, a small amount every day is not only harmless but actually beneficial.

Once again, it comes down to how you drink it. For example, red wine is healthier than white wine. This is because red wine has less sugar and more antioxidants. High quality alcohol is better than low quality alcohol.

This is because the cheap stuff usually adds sulfites and sugar in order to mask the bad flavor and help you get drunk more quickly (so that you are too drunk to care about the taste). These sugars and sulfites are bad for your body.

Drinking moderate amounts of high-quality booze (especially red wine) can help lower cholesterol by raising your HDL (good) cholesterol.

One study has even shown that people who drank 2 to 3 glasses of wine per day (with meals) actually lived longer. Their risk of death was 18% lower than those who did not drink any alcohol at all.

There are a few other health benefits including lowered risk of heart disease, diabetes, and dementia. But remember, these benefits are cancelled out by the health risks of drinking more than 2 or 3 units of alcohol per day. A unit of alcohol is defined as follows:

- 12 ounces of beer
- 5 ounces of wine
- 1.5 ounces of spirits

Also keep in mind that quality counts. If you want the health benefits, skip past the boxed wine and go for a nice bottle of cabernet sauvignon or pinot noir.

Price doesn't always guarantee quality but, in general, try to stick in the mid to high range alcohols (whether it's wine, beer, or spirits). The higher price will be set off by the slow pace at which you drink it (less than 3 units per day will help a good bottle last longer).

Myth #9: Margarine is healthier than butter

Stay away from margarine. It is often marketed as a healthy substitute to butter but it actually is less healthy. While vegetable-based oils (the main ingredient in margarine) *would* be healthy for you because of their high unsaturated fat content, the process of making margarine converts those healthy unsaturated fats into extremely harmful trans fats.

While it is true that margarine tends to contain less cholesterol than butter, this health benefit is entirely offset by the trans fats. It is better to use to use butter than margarine.

At the same time, you should moderate the amount of butter in your diet. Moderate amounts of butter are far better than *any* amount of margarine.

Myth #10: Red meats are dangerous

By now you have probably noticed a general trend in these health myths. Any extreme claims that demonize an entire food group are usually false and all whole, unprocessed foods are good for you (in moderation). This all speaks to the need to maintain *balance* and *variety* in your diet as well as stay away from processed foods.

Red meat is another one of those foods whose bad reputation is grossly undeserved. Pork and beef are full of protein and a wide range of vitamins.

Eating red meat only becomes unhealthy when you eat large amounts of it every single day. This is why it was suggested above that you get your protein from a variety of sources rather than just eating one food to meet all your protein requirements.

"Too much" red meat is roughly defined as anything above 3 ounces of red meat per day or 18 ounces per week. If you keep your consumption below that, then the health benefits of red meat are numerous. Calorie for calorie, red meat packs the most nutrients in the fewest amount of calories. This means it helps you feel satisfied on less calories.

It also contains a high amount of B12 which your body needs in order to build and maintain DNA. B12 is only found in animal products (because plants don't produce it) and some of the highest levels are found in pork and beef (red meat). It also contains the form of iron that is easiest for our body to absorb.

So, there's no reason to banish burgers, steaks, pork chops, or any of your other favorite red meat dishes. Just make sure you are eating them in moderation and that you combine different sources of protein into your diet.

4 Sample Weekly Meal Plans

Now that you know the basics of nutrition including the 5 rules of healthy eating for weight loss and the truth behind the top 10 healthy myths, it's time to start planning your new healthy and delicious eating habits.

The best way to make sure you eat a healthy and varied diet is to plan ahead. Plan your menu at least one week in advance, including breakfasts, lunches, and dinners (and any snacks).

By doing this, you'll make shopping easier because you know exactly what ingredients (and how much of each) you need to buy for the coming week. This helps you cut down on wasteful shopping. Don't buy 5 pounds of apples if your menu only calls for 2 pounds.

It also gives you the chance to cook all your meals ahead and then just freeze them so that during the week, when you come home from work too tired to cook, all you have to do is pull a meal out of the freezer and reheat it.

Week #1

	Sun	Mon	Tues	Wed	Thurs	Fri	Sat
B	Mixed Berries & Yogurt Smoothie	Mixed Berries & Yogurt Smoothie	Mixed Berries & Yogurt Smoothie	Mixed Berries & Yogurt Smoothie	Mixed Berries & Yogurt Smoothie	Mixed Berries & Yogurt Smoothie	Mixed Berries & Yogurt Smoothie
L	Grilled Whole Wheat Pizza	Grilled Whole Wheat Pizza	Last Night's Leftovers	Last Night's Leftovers	Last Night's Leftovers	Last Night's Leftovers	Next Level Chili con Carne
D	Quinoa with Veggies & Eggs	Yellow Curry	One Pot Meatball & Bean Stew	Quinoa with Veggies & Eggs	BBQ Baked Beans with Sweet Potatoes	Yellow Curry	BBQ Baked Beans with Sweet Potatoes
S	Smoothie	Natural Peanut Butter & Honey on Whole Grain Bread	Natural Peanut Butter & Honey on Whole Grain Bread	Natural Peanut Butter & Honey on Whole Grain Bread	Natural Peanut Butter & Honey on Whole Grain Bread	Natural Peanut Butter & Honey on Whole Grain Bread	Smoothie

Week #2

	Sun	Mon	Tues	Wed	Thurs	Fri	Sat
B	Banana, Peanut Butter & Yogurt Smoothie	Banana, Peanut Butter & Yogurt Smoothie	Banana, Peanut Butter & Yogurt Smoothie	Banana, Peanut Butter & Yogurt Smoothie	Banana, Peanut Butter & Yogurt Smoothie	Banana, Peanut Butter & Yogurt Smoothie	Banana, Peanut Butter & Yogurt Smoothie
L	Grilled Whole Wheat Pizza	Grilled Whole Wheat Pizza	Last Night's Leftovers	Last Night's Leftovers	Last Night's Leftovers	Last Night's Leftovers	Next Level Chili con Carne
D	One Pot Meatball & Bean Stew	Baked Spinach & Ricotta Chicken	BBQ Baked Beans with Sweet Potatoes	Quinoa with Veggies & Eggs	One Pot Meatball & Bean Stew	Baked Spinach & Ricotta Chicken	BBQ Baked Beans with Sweet Potatoes
S	Smoothie	Assorted Nuts & Dried Fruits	Assorted Nuts & Dried Fruits	Assorted Nuts & Dried Fruits	Assorted Nuts & Dried Fruits	Assorted Nuts & Dried Fruits	Smoothie

Week #3

	Sun	Mon	Tues	Wed	Thurs	Fri	Sat
B	Spinach, Berries, Almond meal & Yogurt Smoothie	Spinach, Berries, Almond meal & Yogurt Smoothie	Spinach, Berries, Almond meal & Yogurt Smoothie	Spinach, Berries, Almond meal & Yogurt Smoothie	Spinach, Berries, Almond meal & Yogurt Smoothie	Spinach, Berries, Almond meal & Yogurt Smoothie	Spinach, Berries, Almond meal & Yogurt Smoothie
L	Next Level Chili con Carne	Last Night's Leftovers	Last Night's Leftovers	Last Night's Leftovers	Last Night's Leftovers	Grilled Whole Wheat Pizza	Last Night's Leftovers
D	Buffalo Chickpea Macaroni & Cheese	Yellow Curry	Baked Spinach & Ricotta Chicken	Hearty Chicken & Veggie Couscous	Buffalo Chickpea Macaroni & Cheese	Yellow Curry	Hearty Chicken & Veggie Couscous
S	Smoothie	Spinach, Avocado & Strawberry Salad	Spinach, Avocado & Strawberry Salad	Spinach, Avocado & Strawberry Salad	Spinach, Avocado & Strawberry Salad	Spinach, Avocado & Strawberry Salad	Smoothie

Week #4

	Sun	Mon	Tues	Wed	Thurs	Fri	Sat
B	Spinach, Banana, Peach, Orange & Yogurt Smoothie	Spinach, Banana, Peach, Orange & Yogurt Smoothie	Spinach, Banana, Peach, Orange & Yogurt Smoothie	Spinach, Banana, Peach, Orange & Yogurt Smoothie	Spinach, Banana, Peach, Orange & Yogurt Smoothie	Spinach, Banana, Peach, Orange & Yogurt Smoothie	Spinach, Banana, Peach, Orange & Yogurt Smoothie
L	Next Level Chili con Carne	Last Night's Leftovers	Last Night's Leftovers	Last Night's Leftovers	Last Night's Leftovers	Last Night's Leftovers	Grilled Whole Wheat Pizza
D	Sweet Potato Shepherd Pie	Buffalo Chickpea Macaroni & Cheese	Yellow Curry	Hearty Chicken & Veggie Couscous	Sweet Potato Shepherd Pie	Buffalo Chickpea Macaroni & Cheese	Hearty Chicken & Veggie Couscous
S	Smoothie	Cottage Cheese & Peaches	Cottage Cheese & Peaches	Cottage Cheese & Peaches	Cottage Cheese & Peaches	Cottage Cheese & Peaches	Smoothie

You can use these sample menus exactly as written or change them up to suit your own tastes. Don't be afraid to experiment and try out new recipes each week to increase variety and see what kinds of foods and cooking methods you like best.

The recipes for the lunch and dinner meals can all be found below.

Delicious and Nutritious Recipes to Get You Inspired

Here you'll find 10 delicious new recipes to try along with the nutrition information for the key macronutrients (protein, fiber, healthy fats) and a list of other vitamins and minerals that each dish contains.

Once again, thank you for reading this book, and I hope you're getting a lot of valuable information. I would greatly appreciate it if you could take 30 seconds to leave me a review for this book on Amazon.com.

Buffalo Chickpea Macaroni and Cheese

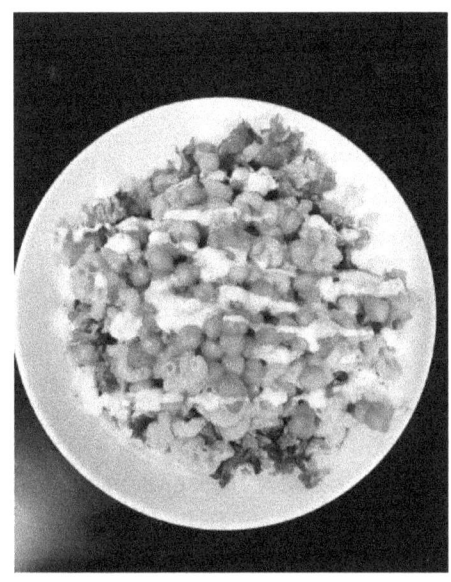

Protein	219 g
Carbohydrates (Fiber)	304 g (52 g)
Fats (Unsaturated)	174 g (63 g)
Key Vitamins & Minerals: Vitamin A, Vitamin C, Vitamin D, B Vitamins, Calcium, Iron, Magnesium, Manganese, Phosphorus, Potassium, Selenium, Zinc	

Ingredients

- 2 cans chickpeas, drained
- ½ cup buffalo sauce
- Drizzle of ranch dressing
- 1 pound dry elbow or shell pasta
- 1 ¼ cups low sodium chicken broth
- 1 ½ cups whole milk

- 2 garlic cloves, minced
- 2 Tbsp. plain Greek yogurt
- 1 tsp salt
- 1 tsp black pepper
- 1 cup shredded cheddar cheese
- 1 cup shredded Gouda cheese
- 1 cup shredded Mozzarella
- ¼ - ½ cup shredded parmesan

Directions

1. Preheat oven to 375° F. Pour chickpeas into a bowl, add buffalo sauce and toss until chickpeas are evenly coated. Line a baking sheet with wax paper or parchment paper. Spread chickpeas across the sheet. Bake for 12 minutes.

2. Remove from oven and roll them with a spoon to turn the bottom sides up. Bake for another 12 minutes or until evenly crispy. Remove from oven, pour into bowl and add another 1 or 2 Tbsp. buffalo sauce. Toss to coat them. Set aside. Leave oven on at same temperature. Boil your pasta according to instructions on package.

3. In a medium saucepan, combine chicken broth, milk, and garlic. Bring to a boil and then immediately reduce heat. Let it simmer for about 15-20 minutes.

4. Pour your broth and milk mixture into a food processor or blender. Add Greek yogurt, salt, and pepper. Blend until smooth. Pour this mixture into a bowl. Add in your cheeses a little at a time until they are all melted. Fold in your cooked pasta. Mix until pasta is evenly coated.

5. Use a paper towel to evenly coat a large baking dish with olive oil. Pour your macaroni and cheese into the dish. Bake

in preheated oven for about 25 minutes. Remove, spoon into serving bowls and top with your buffalo chickpeas. Drizzle a small amount of ranch over the top and serve—or scarf it all down yourself!

BBQ Baked Beans with Sweet Potatoes

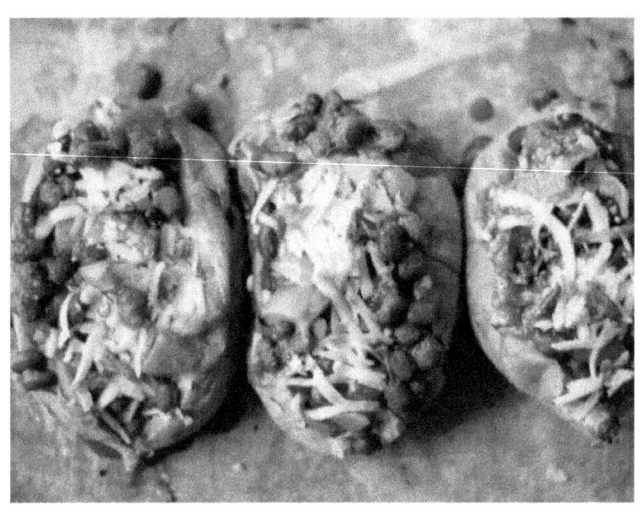

Protein	110 g
Carbohydrates (Fiber)	373 g (94 g)
Fats (Unsaturated)	26 g (16 g)
Key Vitamins & Minerals: Vitamin A, Vitamin C, B Vitamins, Vitamin E, Calcium, Iron, Magnesium, Manganese, Phosphorous, Potassium, Selenium, Zinc	

Ingredients

- 2 purple onions
- 2 garlic cloves
- 1 fresh red chili
- 2 carrots
- 1 heaping tsp paprika
- 1 heaping tsp cumin seeds
- 1 heaping tsp crushed red chili
- 6 sweet potatoes
- 24 oz. tomato paste

- 2 cans beans (assorted varieties)
- ¼ cup BBQ sauce
- ½ cup cheddar cheese, shredded
- 1 cup whole wheat croutons
- Olive oil
- Greek yogurt

Directions

1. Preheat the oven to 350° F. Finely slice the garlic, onion, and chilies together. Place them in a large saucepan over medium heat. Add a few splashes of olive oil. Stir in the paprika, cumin, and crushed red chili. Cook until soft (about 20 minutes). Stir regularly.

2. Wash sweet potatoes and then rub a little olive oil, salt, and pepper over them. Place them on a baking sheet. Set aside. Add tomato paste to your onions, chilies, and garlic. Add a splash of water to the empty tomato paste jar/can. Swirl it around to clean the sides. Pour it into your mixture along with your beans.

3. Drizzle the BBQ sauce in. Add salt and pepper. Stir well. Pour mixture into a large baking dish. Let bake in the oven for about 1 hour. Also place the sweet potatoes in the oven for about the same amount of time.

4. About 20 minutes before it's finished, remove the beans, sprinkle bread crumbs and grated cheddar over the top and return to the lowest shelf of the oven until crispy and golden.

5. Remove beans and sweet potatoes from oven. Place 1 sweet potato per plate. Slice each open and pour a heaping helping of baked beans over it. Add a dollop of Greek yogurt to the top and serve.

6. (Optional): goes well with a simple green salad on the side for some refreshing crunch.

Next Level Chili con Carne

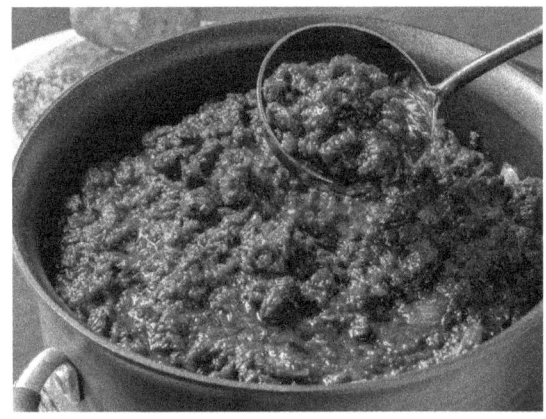

Protein	392 g
Carbohydrates (Fiber)	272 g (63 g)
Fats (Unsaturated)	183 g (81 g)
Key Vitamins & Minerals: Vitamin A, Vitamin C, B Vitamins, Vitamin E, Vitamin K, Calcium, Iron, Magnesium, Manganese, Phosphorus, Potassium, Selenium, Zinc	

Ingredients

- 4 pounds' beef brisket, sliced into 1" pieces
- 2 cups coffee, freshly brewed
- 3 large dry poblano chilies
- 2 heaping tsp paprika
- 2 heaping tsp ground cumin
- 1 heaping tsp oregano
- 2 bay leaves
- 2 purple onions, diced
- 3 or 4 poblano chilies (fresh)
- 2 cinnamon sticks
- 10 garlic cloves, thin slices

- 2 cans beans (kidney, lima, or black)
- 3 bell peppers, seeded and sliced
- 3 Tbsp. molasses
- 4 cans diced tomatoes
- Salt and Pepper (to taste)
- Olive oil
- Sour cream (optional)

Directions

1. Start your coffee brewing while you carefully trim the fat from your brisket and slice into pieces. Soak the dried chilis in your fresh, hot coffee to rehydrate. Put a large baking dish over low heat on the stove. Add a few good splashes of olive oil. Then sprinkle in the oregano, cumin, paprika, onions, and bay leaves. Fry for 10 minutes until onions are soft.

2. Chop up your fresh chilies. Remove dried chilies from the coffee and add to the onion mixture along with half of your fresh chilies. Add cinnamon sticks, garlic, salt, pepper, and a splash of the coffee you used to soak the chilies. Stir well.

3. Add the rest of the coffee, tomatoes, and molasses. Stir. Add in the brisket pieces along with a pinch of salt and pepper. Cover the dish with a lid. Let simmer for about 3 hours. Stir occasionally.

4. After about 2 ½ hours, use forks to pull apart the meat. Add the rest of your fresh chilies. Add beans. Let this simmer for about 30 minutes without the lid on. Stir occasionally. Serve in a bowl or over rice. Add a dollop of sour cream before serving.

5. (Optional) this dish goes well with a really fresh, tangy salad on the side.

Quinoa Topped with Veggies and Eggs

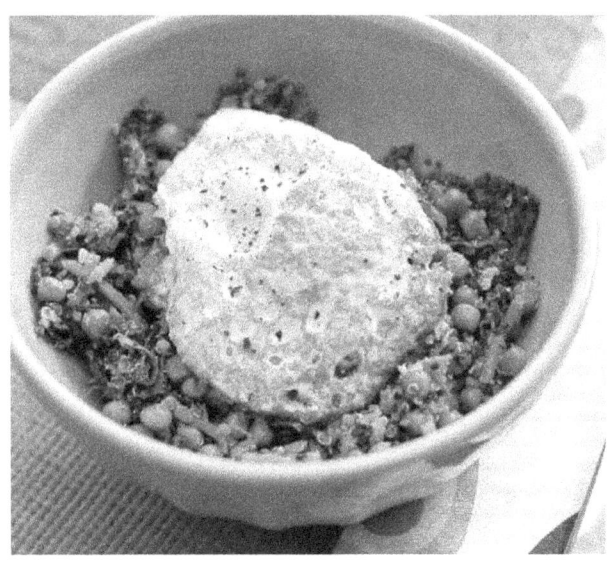

Protein	84 g
Carbohydrates (Fiber)	172 g (44 g)
Fats (Unsaturated)	57 g (27 g)
Key Vitamins & Minerals: Vitamin A, Vitamin C, B Vitamins, Vitamin E, Vitamin K, Calcium, Iron, Magnesium, Manganese, Phosphorus, Potassium, Selenium, Zinc	

Ingredients

- ½ pound quinoa
- 1 pinch of cumin seeds
- 1 can black beans
- 1 fresh red chili, sliced finely
- 1 fresh jalapeno, sliced finely
- 2 Tbsp. white wine vinegar
- 1 pinch of sugar
- Juice of ½ a lemon

- 6 large eggs
- 1 avocado
- 1 tomato, sliced
- ½ pound cherry tomatoes, quartered
- 2 spring onions, sliced finely
- 1 small bunch fresh mint
- 1 small bunch fresh parsley
- Salt and Pepper (to taste)
- Olive oil
- Hot chili sauce

Directions

1. Cook the quinoa according to instructions on the package. Add a pinch of salt while cooking. Add a couple splashes of olive oil to a frying pan and place over high heat.

2. Once hot, add the cumin seeds and fry for about 30 seconds. Add beans and a pinch of salt. Cook for about 5 to 10 minutes (until beans are crispy). While the beans cook, put your sliced chilies in a bowl. Add vinegar, sugar, and a pinch of salt. Set aside.

3. Drain the quinoa then drizzle on olive oil and lemon juice. Spread it out on a tray. Set aside. Pour the cooked beans into a bowl. Wipe the pan clean (don't rinse). Add a splash of olive oil and return to medium heat.

4. Once hot, crack the eggs into the frying pan and cook to your liking. For the perfect sunny side up eggs, you just need 3 or 4 minutes. Layer the eggs on top of the quinoa. Then spoon the beans over it. Sprinkle the tomatoes, spring onions, and chilies over the top and drizzle in a little of the vinegar mixture the chilies were soaking in.

5. Halve the avocado and remove the pit. Scoop out small spoonfuls of the avocado flesh and drop them all across the top. Roughly chop the mint and parsley. Sprinkle it on. Add a drizzle of olive oil and however much hot chili sauce you like. Finally, dish this out onto plates and serve.

One Pot Meatball & Bean Stew

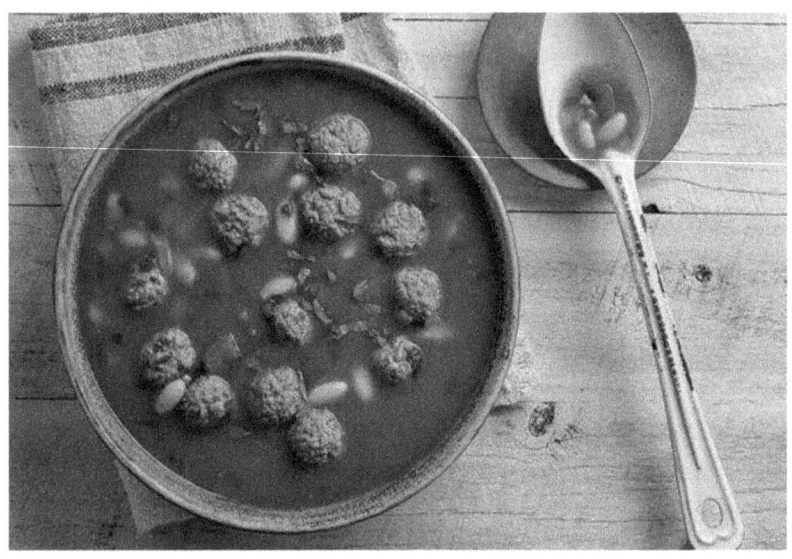

Protein	114 g
Carbohydrates (Fiber)	119 g (27 g)
Fats (Unsaturated)	46 g (21 g)
Key Vitamins & Minerals: Vitamin A, Vitamin C, B Vitamins, Vitamin E, Vitamin K, Calcium, Iron, Magnesium, Manganese, Phosphorus, Potassium, Selenium, Zinc	

Ingredients

- ¾ pound ground pork (or beef, lamb, turkey, etc.)
- 2 tsp olive oil
- 1 purple onion, chopped
- 2 Jalapeños, sliced (or preferred pepper)
- 3 garlic cloves, minced
- 1 Tbsp. smoked paprika
- 2 cans diced tomatoes
- 1 can lima beans

- 2 tsp sugar
- 1 small bunch parsley, chopped roughly

Directions

1. Heat olive oil in a large pan over medium high heat. Work the seasonings into the pork with your hands and shape it into small meatballs. Add the meatballs to the pan and cook for about 5 minutes (or until golden brown all over). Push all the meatballs to one side of the pan.

2. Add onions and jalapeños. Cook for another 5 minutes. Stir occasionally. Stir in the garlic and paprika. Push the meatballs back into the rest of the pan and stir together for a minute or so.

3. Add the tomatoes. Cover with a lid and let simmer for about 10 minutes. Add the beans, sugar, and seasonings. Let simmer without the lid for another 10 minutes. Spoon into bowls. Top with fresh, chopped parsley and serve.

4. (Optional): This is great with a slice of warm, crusty bread or cornbread for dunking in and soaking up the juices. Add a fresh strawberry, walnut, spinach salad on the side to round out the meal.

Sweet Potato Shepherd's Pie

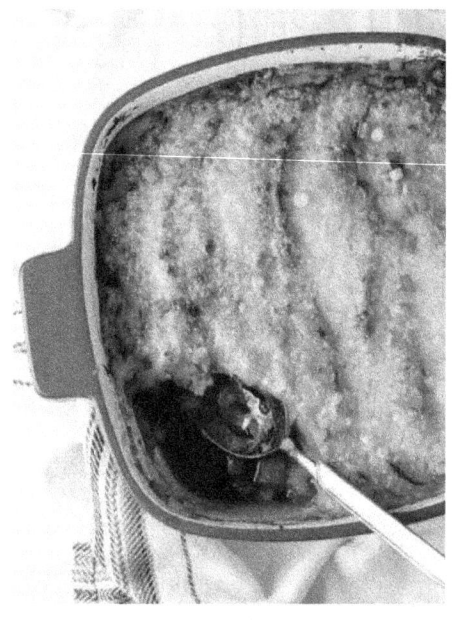

Protein	144 g
Carbohydrates (Fiber)	319 g (64 g)
Fats (Unsaturated)	77 g (35.5 g)
Key Vitamins & Minerals: Vitamin A, Vitamin C, B Vitamins, Vitamin E, Calcium, Iron, Magnesium, Manganese, Phosphorus, Potassium, Selenium, Zinc	

Ingredients

- 1 Tbsp. olive oil
- 2 yellow onions, chopped finely
- 2 garlic cloves, chopped
- 2 carrots, grated
- 2 Tbsp. thyme
- 1 pound extra lean ground beef (or turkey, lamb, etc.)

- 1 ½ cups red lentils
- ½ pound turnips, diced
- 2 Tbsp. plain flour
- 3 ¼ cups low sodium beef stock
- ¾ cup red wine
- 2 pounds' sweet potatoes, diced
- 1 ½ cups plain Greek yogurt

Directions

1. Preheat the oven to 350° F. Heat olive oil in a large pan over high heat. Add the onions and fry until golden (about 6 minutes). Add garlic, carrots, and thyme. Cook for another 4 minutes.

2. Stir in the ground beef. When it is browned, add lentils, turnips, and flour. Cook for 1 or 2 minutes. Slowly pour in the beef stock and the red wine. Cover and let simmer for 35 to 40 minutes.

3. While that's simmering, boil the sweet potatoes until tender (about 15 minutes). Drain and mash with the yogurt, nutmeg, and pepper. Pour the meat mixture into a large baking dish. Spread the sweet potato mash over the top. Put in the oven and let bake for about 1 hour (or until the top starts to brown).

4. (Optional) Serve with a side of broccoli or peas for a complete and satisfying dinner.

Baked Spinach Ricotta Chicken

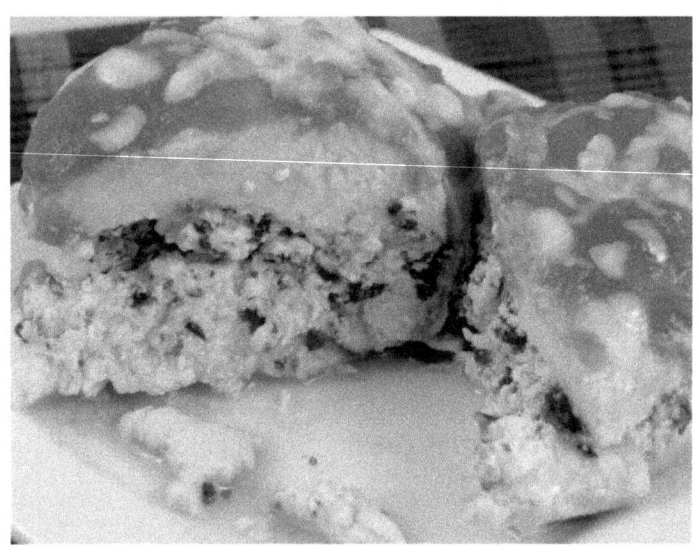

Protein	50 g
Carbohydrates (Fiber)	70 g (31 g)
Fats (Unsaturated)	17 g (5 g)
Key Vitamins & Minerals: Vitamin A, Vitamin C, B Vitamins, Vitamin E, Vitamin K, Calcium, Iron, Magnesium, Manganese, Potassium	

Ingredients

- 3 healthy bunches fresh spinach
- 4 Tbsp. ricotta
- Zest and Juice of 1 Lemon
- Ground nutmeg
- 4 chicken breasts, skinless
- 2 Tbsp. olive oil
- ½ cup seasoned bread crumbs
- 3 Zucchini, cut into thick strips

- 2 Jalapeños, sliced (or other preferred pepper)
- 2 purple onions, cut into wedges
- ½ pound cherry tomatoes
- 4 garlic cloves

Directions

1. Preheat the oven to 375° F. Bring water to a boil in a tea kettle or pot. Place spinach in a large strainer. Pour the boiling water over to wilt the spinach. Let it drain fully.

2. Chop the spinach and put it into a large bowl. Add ricotta, lemon zest, nutmeg, salt, and pepper. Mix it up well. Use a sharp knife to cut a slit into the side of each chicken breast. Slide your fingers in to make a little pocket inside the breast.

3. Spoon in the spinach and ricotta mixture liberally. Rub the breasts with olive oil and press the breadcrumbs into its surface. Place the prepared chicken breasts into a large baking dish (so that none of the pieces are touching).

4. In another baking dish, add the zucchini, tomatoes, jalapeños, onion, and garlic. Liberally drizzle olive oil over them. Add salt and pepper to taste. Place both dishes in the oven and bake for about 30 minutes. Stir the vegetables once in this time.

5. Remove when the chicken is cooked all the way through and the breadcrumbs have turned golden. Remove the garlic cloves from the vegetables, mash with lemon juice. Stir the mixture back into the vegetables. Serve the chicken with a healthy side of your roasted vegetables.

Yellow Curry

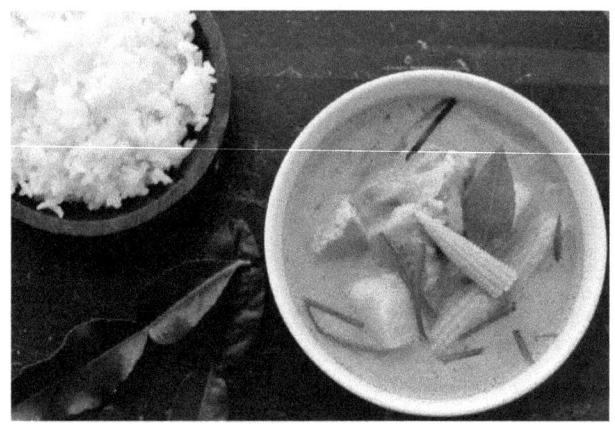

Protein	163 g
Carbohydrates (Fiber)	200 g (27 g)
Fats (Unsaturated)	5 g (4 g)
Key Vitamins & Minerals: Vitamin A, Vitamin C, B Vitamins, Iron, Calcium, Manganese, Potassium, Selenium, Zinc	

Ingredients

- 2 yellow onions
- 4 garlic cloves
- 1 piece of fresh ginger, 1" – 2" thick
- 2 fresh red chilies
- 1 fresh green chili
- 1 chicken bouillon cube
- 1 tsp honey
- 1 tsp ground turmeric
- 2 tsps. curry powder
- 8 chicken drumsticks
- 1 can chickpeas
- 1 tsp tomato paste

- 1 lemon
- 1 ½ cups basmati rice
- Olive oil
- Plain Greek yogurt

Directions

1. Put the garlic, ginger, 2 red chilies, and 1 onion in a food processor. Crumble in the bouillon cube. Add the honey and spices. Place the lid on and blend into a paste.

2. Put a large baking dish over medium high heat on the stove. Add a few splashes of oil. Remove the skins from the drumsticks. Once the dish is heated, fry the chicken until they turn golden (about 10 minutes). Turn the drumsticks occasionally with tongs. Remove drumsticks, put them on a plate.

3. Chop the remaining onion and green chili roughly. Add to the pan and let cook until softened. Bring 2 ½ cups of water to a boil. Spoon in the paste and let cook for about 5 minutes. Pour in the boiling water. Drain the chickpeas and add them in. Add in the tomato paste and a pinch of salt and pepper. Stir well.

4. Put the chicken back in the pan. Place the lid on. Reduce the heat to medium low or low and let simmer for about 45 minutes. 15 minutes before it's ready, add rice to a saucepan with 3 cups of water. Add a pinch of salt and drizzle in some olive oil. Bring it to a boil.

5. Once boiling, reduce heat to low and let simmer until all liquid has been absorbed (about 12 minutes). Spoon the rice onto the plate and top with a drumstick and plenty of curry sauce. Add a dollop of yogurt.

Hearty Chicken & Veggie Couscous

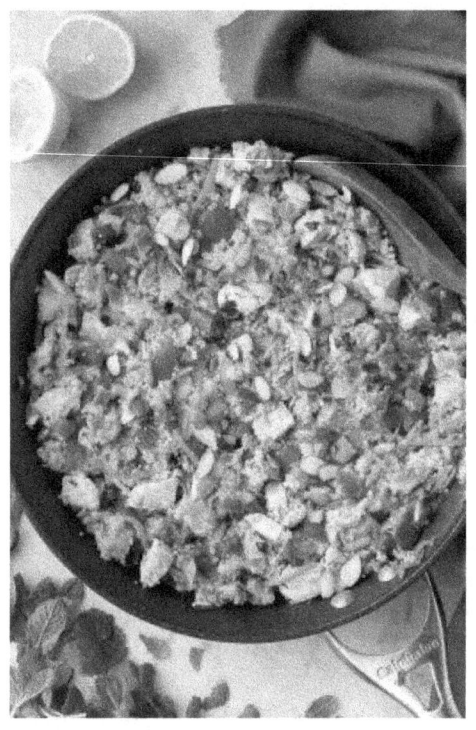

Protein	111 g
Carbohydrates (Fiber)	130 g (20.5 g)
Fats (Unsaturated)	60 g (36 g)
Key Vitamins & Minerals: Vitamin A, Vitamin C, B Vitamins, Potassium, Iron, Magnesium, Selenium, Zinc	

Ingredients

- 3 Zucchini
- 3 Carrots
- 3 purple onions
- ½ pound mushrooms (quartered)
- Whole cherry tomatoes (to taste)

- 6 garlic cloves, peeled
- 4 Tbsp. olive oil
- 3 tsp paprika
- 5 tsp crushed red chili
- 6 chicken thighs, skin on (or breasts)
- ½ cup couscous
- Fresh parsley or mint, chopped roughly
- Sweet chili sauce (optional)

Directions

1. Preheat the oven to 375° F. Chop vegetables into small chunks. Chop onion into wedges. Place on a baking sheet with the garlic cloves. Drizzle olive oil over the top. Sprinkle a dash or two of salt and pepper. Set aside. Sprinkle salt, pepper, paprika, and crushed red chili over the chicken thighs. Rub the seasonings into the skin.

2. Put the chicken thighs in with the vegetables. Nestle them in together. Place dish in the oven and let roast until the vegetables get crispy and the chicken is cooked through (about 30 minutes).

3. About 15 minutes before it's ready, bring water to a boil on the stove. Pour the dry couscous into a bowl. Pour the boiling water over it. Cover the bowl with plastic wrap and set aside.

4. Mix the couscous with a fork to separate the grains. Toss the vegetables in the bowl of couscous with the fresh mint or parsley. Add a dash of salt and pepper. Scoop out a helping of couscous and veggies onto a plate. Top with a chicken thigh. Drizzle on sweet chili sauce (to taste). Serve.

Grilled Whole Wheat Pizza

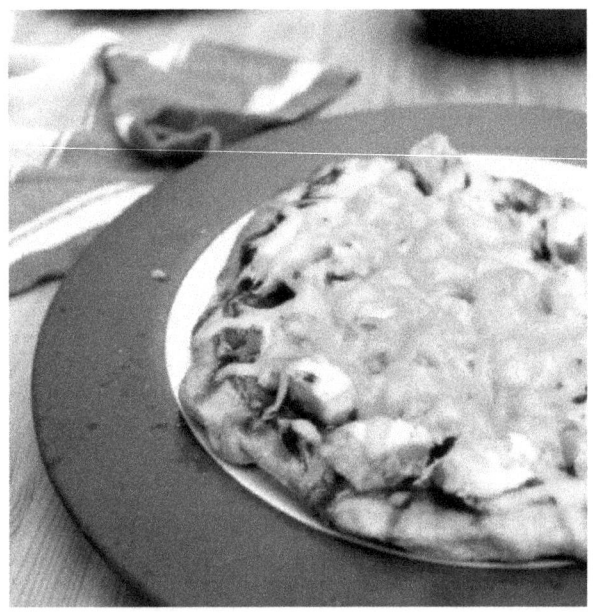

Protein	29 g
Carbohydrates (Fiber)	182 g (18 g)
Fats (Unsaturated)	3 g (1.5 g)
Key Vitamins & Minerals: B vitamins, Iron, Selenium	

* Nutrition values for pizza crust only

Ingredients

- 1 cup whole grain flour
- 1 cup all purpose, unbleached flour
- 1 package (2 ¼ tsp) quick rising yeast
- 1 tsp salt
- ½ tsp sugar
- ¾ cup hot water (120° F to 130° F)
- 1 Tbsp. olive oil

- Sauce of your choice
- Toppings of your choice

Directions

1. Combine the whole grain flour with the all-purpose flour, yeast, salt, and sugar. Blend together thoroughly. In a measuring cup, combine hot water with oil. Blend into the flour until it becomes a sticky ball. The dough should be quite soft. If it seems dry, add warm water 1 or 2 Tbsp. at a time. If too sticky, add flour 1 or 2 Tbsp. at a time.

2. Blend until it becomes a ball of dough. Then knead for a couple minutes. Place the dough on a lightly floured surface. Cover with a clean, damp cloth. Let rest 10 to 20 minutes. Roll the dough out until it's about 1" – 2" inches thick. Add sauce and toppings as desired. Experiment with different creative combinations!

3. Put the pizza on the grill until crust becomes crispy and golden and the cheese is melted (about 10 to 15 minutes). If you don't want to use the grill (or don't have one), preheat your oven to 500° F and bake until ready (about 10 to 15 minutes).

Others who are considering purchasing this book would love to know what you think. If you could spare a few seconds, they would greatly appreciate reading an honest review from you. Simply visit the page on Amazon.com.

15-Minute Workouts

15-Minute Beginner Back Workouts

This chapter contains your first 3 sets of complete workouts. So, let's get to it!

We'll start with a quick 10-minute warm up routine. You can use this same warm up to start each of the 3 workouts in this chapter.

You'll also get a 10-minute cool down routine at the end, which can also be used after all 3 workouts.

Warm ups and cool downs are absolutely essential. If you just jump right into a workout without giving your muscles time to warm up, you are putting yourself at risk for sprains, tears, cramps, joint damage, and all kinds of painful injuries that could end up leaving you bed ridden for weeks.

No matter how excited you are to start these back-sculpting exercises; the warm up is absolutely essential.

The same goes for cool downs. This 10-minute portion mostly consists of stretching and sometimes light cardio.

The stretching helps keep your freshly worked muscles flexible and smooth, which prevents post-workout cramping and helps increase muscle growth.

As you learned in the previous chapter, muscle growth isn't just important for toning and shaping your body, it's also essential for burning fat.

10 Minute Warm Up

For your first warm up of the book, let's start with swimming. Of course, you can do any cardio activity you like for a warm up but this is just to give you an idea. Jump in the pool and swim at an easy pace for 3 minutes.

Then, bump up the intensity a tiny bit for the next 2 minutes. Then, go back to your original intensity for the next 2 minutes. Finally, swim at a higher intensity (faster than you have so far but still not so fast that you become exhausted) for the final 3 minutes.

Beginner Back Sculpting Workout #1 (No Equipment)

Do each exercise for 30 seconds. Repeat the full series 6 times for a total of 15 minutes.

1. **Back Extensions**

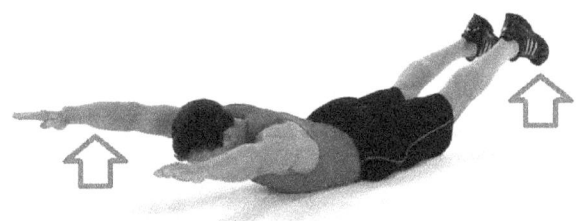

Lie down on your back with your toes pointed toward the wall and your arms above your head, palms on the floor.

Keep your legs and torso straight as you raise both of them off the floor. Bend as much as you can until only your stomach is touching the ground. Hold this for 30 seconds.

2. **Swimmers**

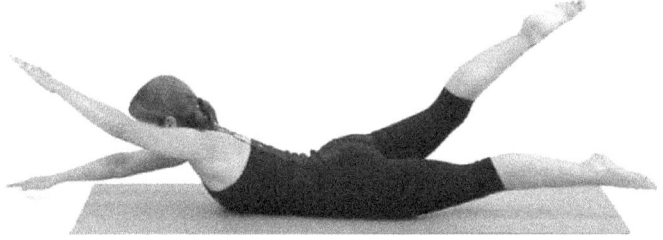

Get into the same position as you did for the first exercise. This time, raise your arms and leg up and down as if you were swimming.

Maintain your form as you do this so that your stomach is the only thing touching the floor. Do this for 30 seconds.

3. Leaning Shoulder Lifts

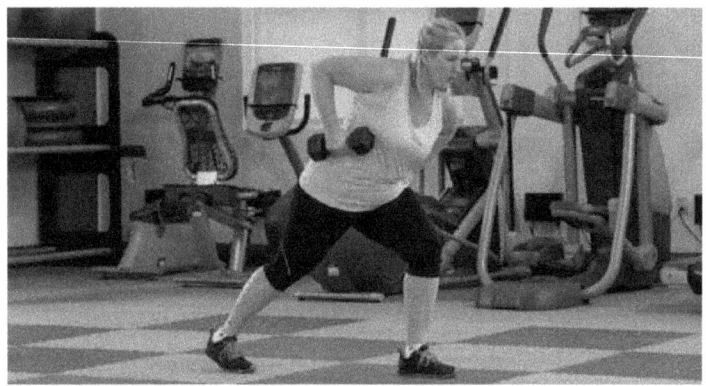

For this and the next 2 exercises, you will need to hold canned food or get small weights. Stand with your legs hip width apart.

Bring your right leg back into a lunge. Lean forward just enough to look down at the floor but don't rest your torso on your front leg. Holding small weights or cans, lift your arms up and down.

Do this for 30 seconds. The next time you do this exercise, put your left leg back. Alternate each time so that each leg does the exercise 3 times.

4. Leaning One Leg Shoulder Lifts

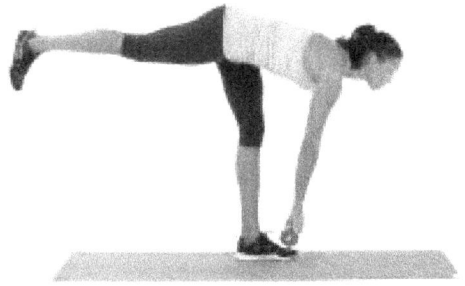

This is similar to the previous exercise except that while you are doing it, your back leg should be elevated off the ground so that you are balancing on just one leg.

Do this for 30 seconds and remember to switch legs each time.

5. *Lat Pullover*

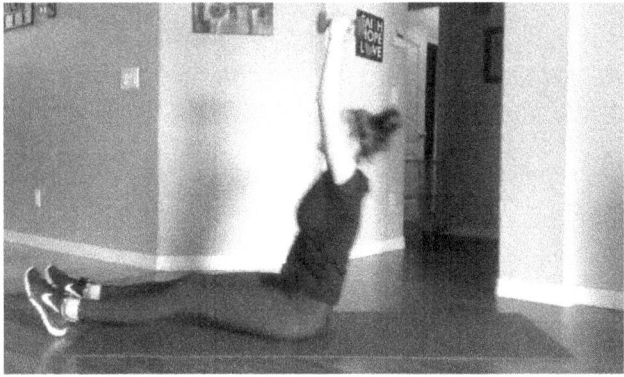

Lie down on your back with your arms above your head. Hold cans or small weights in your hands. Lift your arms up off the ground toward the ceiling and then toward the wall across from you.

As you are lifting your arms, lift your torso up as well into a sit up. Do not move your legs for this exercise.

Continue for 30 seconds.

Beginner Back Sculpting Workout #2 (With Equipment)

Equipment Needed: Resistance Band

Do each exercise for 30 seconds. Repeat the full series 6 times for a total of 15 minutes.

1. **Spread Your Wings**

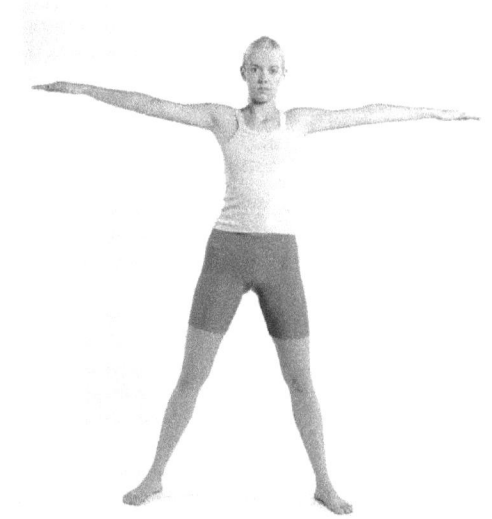

Stand straight with your legs hip width apart. Holding the resistance, spread your arms apart in opposite directions (like wings).

Bring them back to a close in front of you. Continue this or 30 seconds.

2. **Reverse Wings**

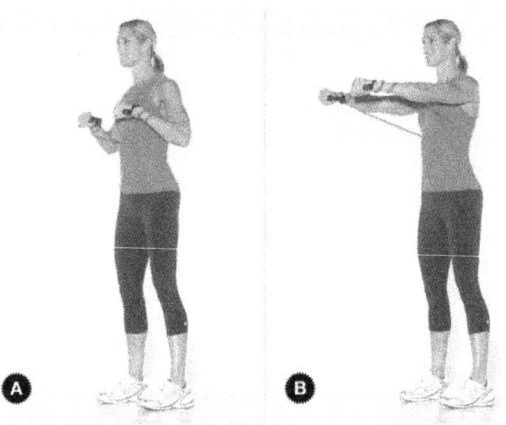

Hold the resistance band so that it is behind your back. Pull your arms together straight out in front of you until your hands touch. Spread your arms back apart. Continue for 30 seconds.

3. *Curls with Resistance Band*

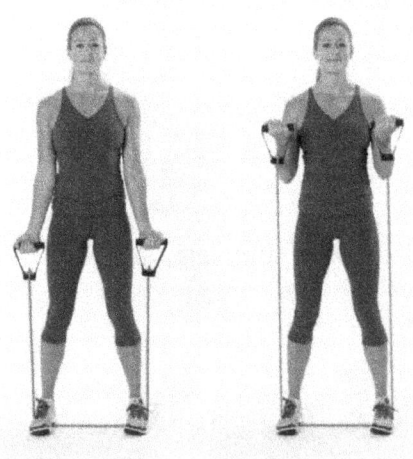

Stand straight with legs just wider than hip width apart. Place the resistance band under both feet and hold one end in each hand.

Keep your feet firmly planted and pull the resistance band up toward the ceiling as high as you can.

Release it back down. Repeat for 30 seconds.

4. *Fencing Lunges*

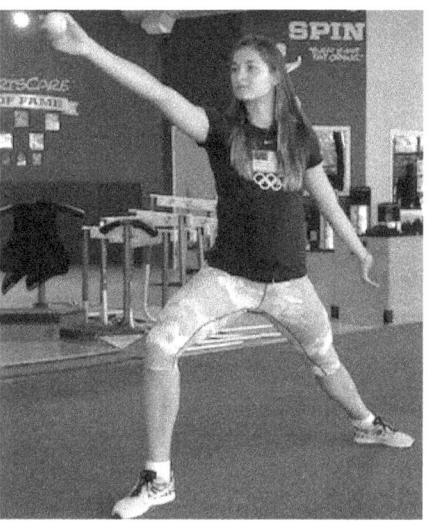

Get into a lunge position. Wrap a resistance band under your front foot so that you are holding it down.

Pull each end with your arms and spread them out into wings (like with the first exercise).

Do this for 30 seconds. Remember to alternate legs each time you do this exercise.

5. *Opposing Arm and Leg Reaches*

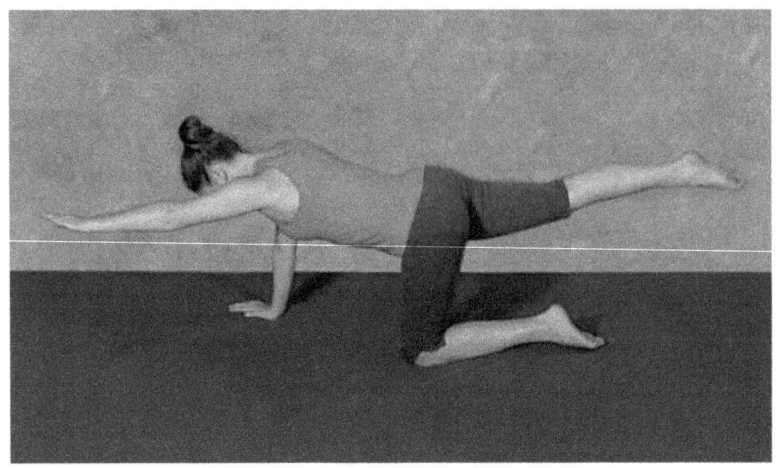

Get down on all fours. Wrap a resistance band around your right foot.

Hold both ends of it with your left hand. Stretch your right foot straight back at the same time that your reach your left arm forward so that you are stretching the resistance band in both directions.

Continue for 30 seconds. Switch arms and legs each time you do the exercise.

Beginner Back Sculpting Workout #3 (Cardio Based)

Option 1:

Rowing

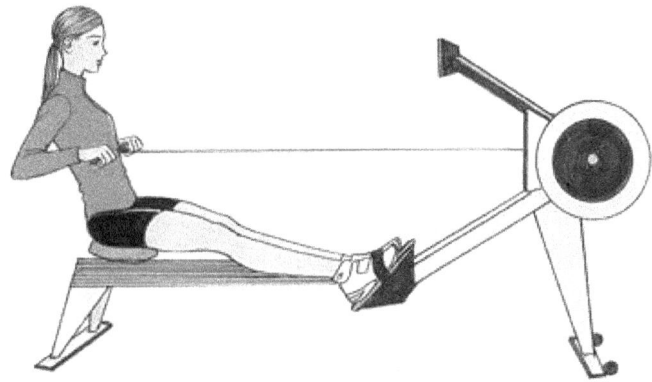

Use a rowing machine or an actual row boat for this exercise. Start with 20 seconds of maximum intensity rowing then slow down to a more moderate pace for 40 seconds.

Continue alternating between these intervals for 15 minutes. As you get better, increase the high intensity interval and decrease the low intensity interval until you get to 40 seconds of high intensity and 20 seconds of low intensity.

Option 2:

Swimming

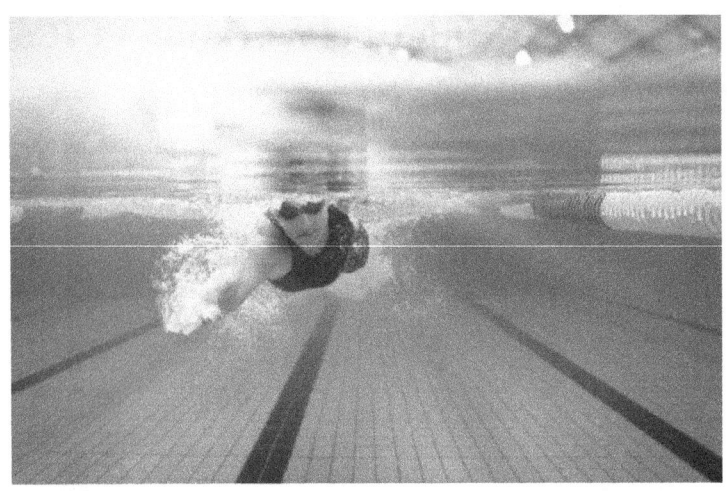

Get in a pool, lake or other body of water where you can swim. Start by swimming as fast as you can for 20 seconds. Then swim at a more moderate speed for 40 seconds.

Continue alternating between these intervals for 15 minutes. As your fitness improves, increase the high intensity interval and decrease the low intensity interval until you can do 40 seconds of high intensity and 20 seconds of low intensity.

10 Minute Cool Down

For this first cool down, you want to start with 5 minutes of light cardio. Swimming, rowing, or even skipping rope will help. If your arms are dead weight after the workout, you can do cardio that uses your legs more (walking, cycling, etc.).

Just go at an easy pace for 5 minutes. Afterward, do 5 minutes of stretching. The cool down routine in chapter 4 will also work perfectly after any of the workouts in this chapter.

15-Minute Advanced Back Workouts

This chapter is for those who want to heat things up and make their workout more challenging. The routines you'll get in this chapter target the back just like the routines you saw in chapter 3. They are just more intense and provide you with a great challenge so that you can keep your body working.

If you can't remember the last time you really exercised, you might want to hold off on these workouts until you've mastered the beginner's level workouts from the previous chapter.

It is important to challenge yourself but you have to know your limits and make sure you don't push yourself to your literal breaking point.

Start with what your body can handle and push yourself a little further each day. Don't just dive right into advanced level workouts without giving your body time to prepare.

Just like in the last chapter, we'll start with a quick 10 minute warm up and end with a 10-minute cool down. These can be used with each of the 3 workout routines in this chapter.

Keep in mind that what you do for your warm up and cool downs is really up to you. If you find the samples here boring or not useful for your needs, change them up to better suit you.

10 Minute Warm Up

For this warm up, you'll do some cardio that focuses on your back and arms. Punch in the air or at a punching bag at a moderate speed for 2 minutes.

Then increase the speed slightly for the next 2 minutes. Increase the speed again for the next 3 minutes. Increase the speed again for the final 3 minutes.

Advanced Back Sculpting Workout #1 (No Equipment)

Do each exercise for 60 seconds. Repeat the full series 3 times to get a total of 15 minutes.

1. *V Crunches*

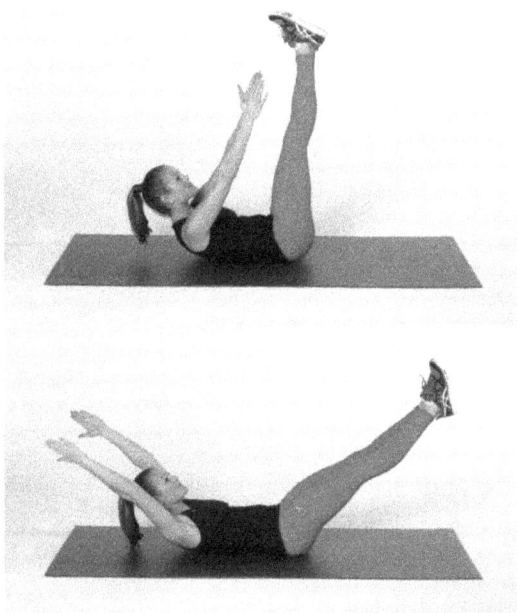

Lie down on your back with your toes point and your arms straight above your head palms facing the ceiling. Keep your toes pointed and your knees straight as your lift your legs up to point at where the wall meets the ceiling.

At the same time, lift your torso up until your body is forming a V shape. Lower your arms so that they are on either side of your thighs and pointing straight at the wall across from you (not holding your legs).

Squeeze your legs and torso up together as far as you can while maintaining balance then lower back into the V shape. Pretend you are a fold up bed trying to close and open. Do this for 60 seconds.

2. *Plank with Leg Bends*

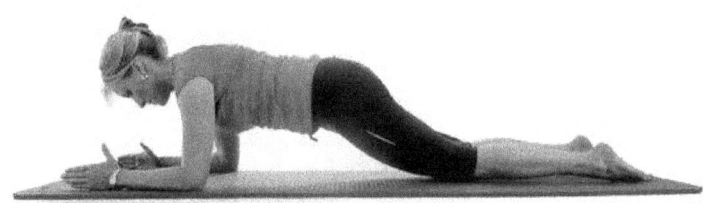

Lie down on your stomach. Lift up onto your elbows so that they form a 90° angle and your palms are flat on the floor.

Lift up into plank position. Lift your right leg up and bend your knee and pull your toes as close to your head as you can. Put your leg back down.

Repeat this with your other leg. Continue alternating for 60 seconds.

3. *Side Plank with Knee Twists*

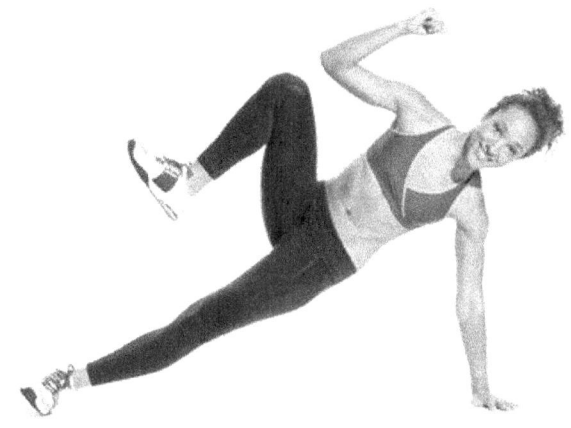

Get into plank position. Carefully twist your full body so that your foot is lying on its outer side and the left side of your body is completely above the right side and you are looking toward the wall.

Hold this position as you bend your left leg up toward your chest then open it up so that your knee is pointing toward the ceiling.

Then, stretch your leg out and up so that your toe is pointing toward the ceiling. Lower your leg back down. Continue doing this for 30 seconds then switch and do the same thing on the other side.

4. *Reclined Corkscrew*

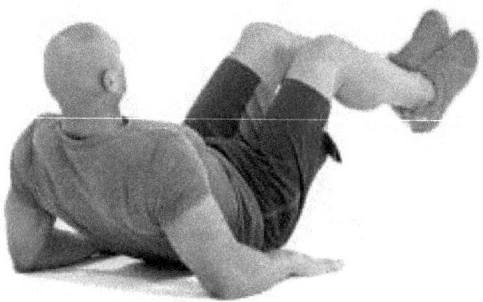

Lie down on your back with your arms at your side, palms on the floor. Keep your legs straight and point your toes as you lift them up to point toward the ceiling.

Lower them down to the right side to point toward the right wall. Swing them around to center and point them at the wall across from you. Then swing them to the other side to point toward the right wall.

Make this one fluid movement of swinging your legs around. Do not allow your back or torso to lift off the floor or move.

5. *Dolphin Sit Ups*

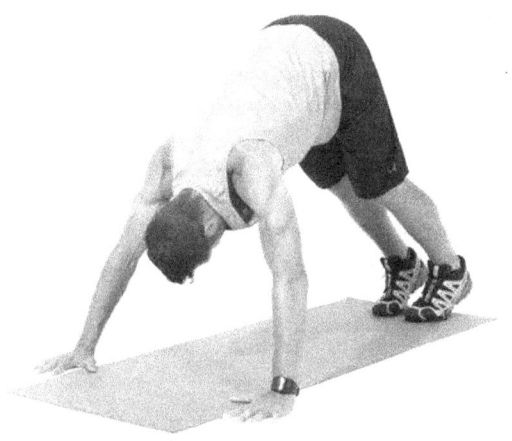

Lie down on your stomach with your arms down by your sides, palms facing up.

Draw your head, shoulders, and torso up and back as far as you can bend. Try to look at the ceiling. Lower yourself back down. Continue this for 60 seconds.

Advanced Back Sculpting Workout #2 (With Equipment)

Equipment Needed: Pull Up Bar

1. Pull Ups

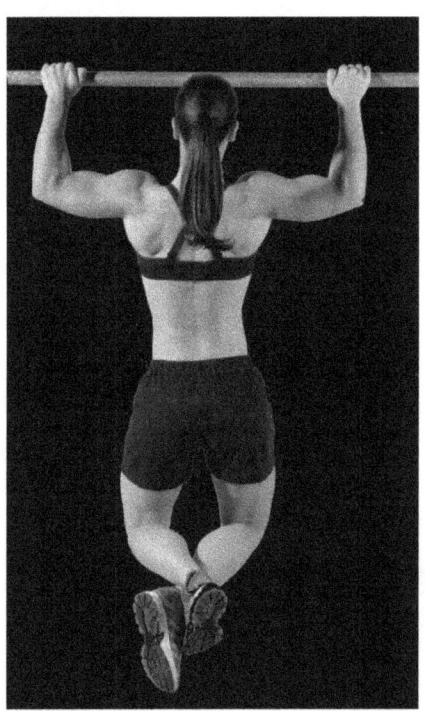

Use a sturdy pull up bar to do as many pull ups as you can in 60 seconds. Pay attention to form and make sure you are doing full pull ups.

That means your head should come in line with the bar.

2. Side to Side Pull Ups

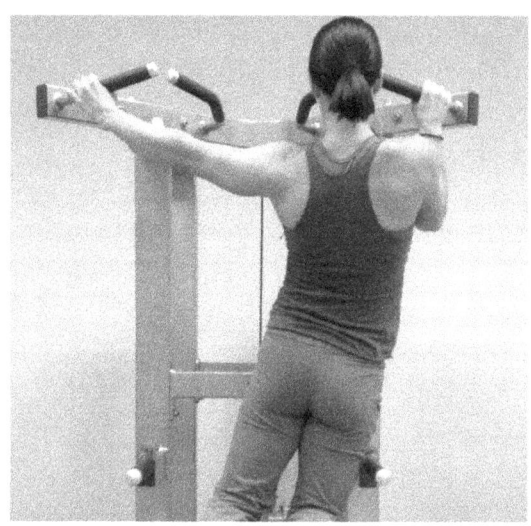

These are like regular pull ups except that instead of just coming straight up to the center, you pull your body to the side at the same time that you are going up so that your nose comes in line with the bar on the outer side of one hand instead of in between.

Continue alternating between pulling up to the left side and the right side as many times as you can for 60 seconds.

3. **Windshield Wipers**

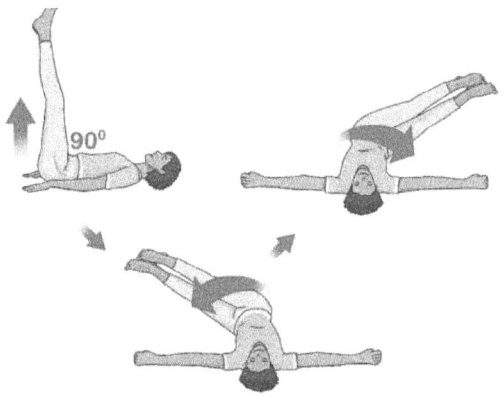

Pull yourself all the way up so that your hips are in line with the bar. Keep your legs together and your knees straight as you lift your legs up and point your toes toward the wall across from you.

Now lift them up higher to point at the ceiling. You will be sort of folded around the bar. Use your hips and lower back to move your legs from side to side as if they were windshield wipers. Do this for 60 seconds.

4. Leg Raises

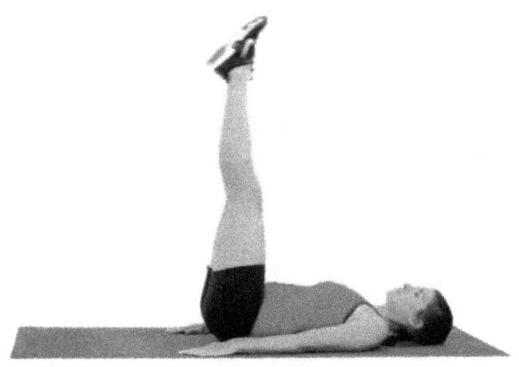

Get into the same position as you were for the windshield wipers. Point your toes toward the wall across from you.

Lower your legs to point toward the floor and then raise them back up to point toward the wall. Continue this for 60 seconds.

5. Chest Dips

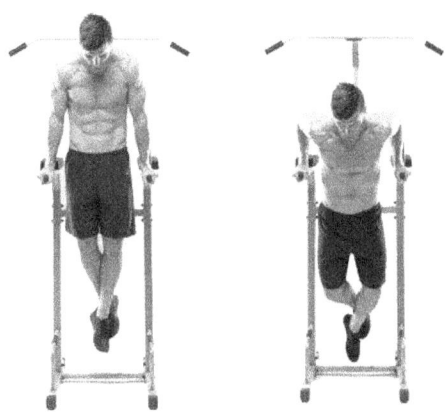

Return again to the position you were in for the previous 2 exercises. Position your hands a little further apart (about 18" to 24" inches apart).

Keep your full body from head to toe flexed and straight. Raise your legs behind you slightly so that your body is at a slight angle.

Bend your elbows and lower your chest down toward the bar. Lift back up. Continue this for 60 seconds.

Advanced Back Sculpting Workout #3 (Cardio Based)

Option 1:

Rowing

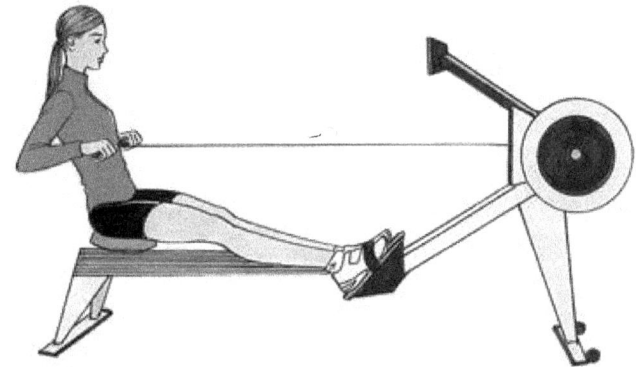

Rowing is an excellent sport that targets and tones your back. You can either use a rowing machine or get in a boat and actually row on a lake.

In either case, do 40 seconds of rowing at your maximum speed and intensity. Then do 20 seconds at a more moderate speed and intensity. Do each interval 15 times for a total of 15 minutes.

Option 2:

Swimming

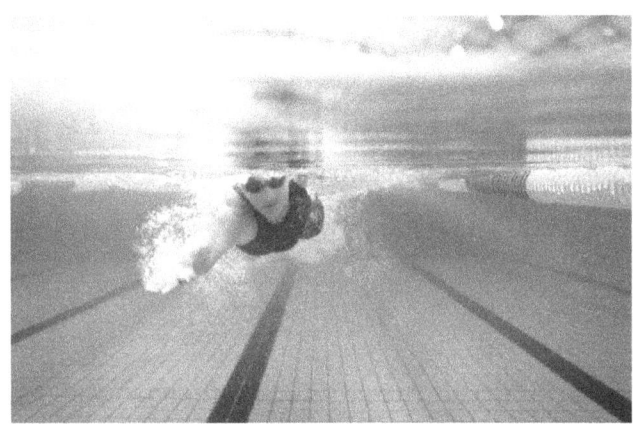

Swimming is a great cardio activity for your back and the rest of your body.

Get into a pool and start swimming laps. Swim for 40 seconds at your maximum speed. Then swim for 20 seconds at a more moderate speed.

You will probably have to count off the seconds in your head since it's not as easy to use a timer in the pool. In this case, you will do each interval 15 times for a total of 15 minutes.

10 Minute Cool Down

Do some form of light cardio for 5 minutes. This can be swimming, rowing, walking, jumping jacks, or anything else that keeps your heart rate elevated.

After 5 minutes of light cardio, you'll need to stretch. Again, we'll focus on the back and arms because they got the most serious workout.

Start by raising your arms over your head and bending your elbows so that your lower arms hang behind your head.

Grab the outside of your right elbow with your left hand and pull it toward your head. You will feel a stretch along your upper arm. As you hold this position, plant your feet firmly on the ground and bend just your torso from left to right slowly.

Your hips and legs should continue to face forward. Only let your torso twist. Do this for 60 seconds. Switch arms and continue for another 60 seconds.

Kneel down so that your shins and the tops of your feet are flat against the floor. Sit down on your calves. Fold your torso over so that your forehead touches the floor.

Clasp your hands together behind your butt and lift them up toward the ceiling as high as they will go. Hold this for 60 seconds.

Unclasp your hands and drop them to the floor.

Bring your right hand under your chest and stick your arm straight out to the other side so that it is completely folded across your chest and your hand is peeking out from your left side.

Let your body weight drop onto your arm. Hold this for 60 seconds. Switch arms and repeat.

Enjoying this book?

Check out my other best sellers!

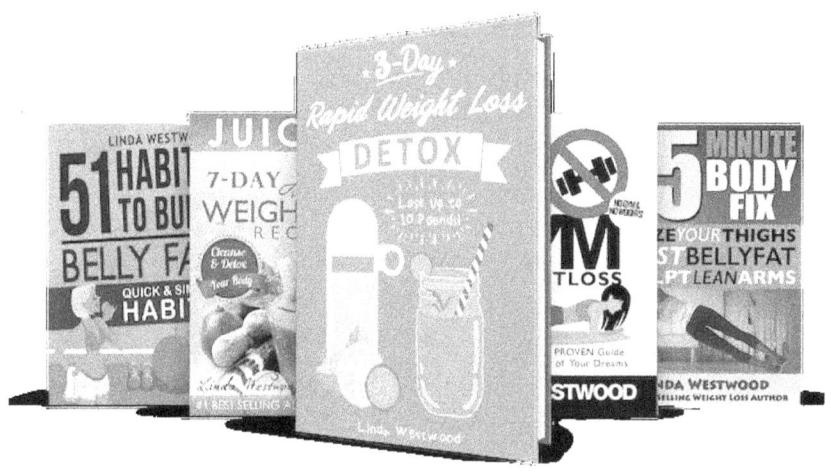

Get your next book on sale here:

TopFitnessAdvice.com/go/books

15-Minute Beginner Butt Workouts

It's time to start getting that butt in shape so that you can flaunt it all summer (and all year) long! If you are new to the world of exercise, you can start with any of these three simple beginner's workouts.

10 Minute Warm Up

As usually, you need to start with a quality 10 minute warm up. Your warm up should be cardio based so that it can really get your heart pumping and get enough oxygen to your muscles that will be ready for the workout ahead.

Your cardio can be anything you enjoy from walking, running, swimming, cycling, or even just skipping rope!

For this warm up, we'll use skipping rope because it's fun cardio activity that wakes up your glutes (butt muscles!) and you can easily do it at home.

Start by skipping rope for 3 minutes at a moderate speed. Remember, the purpose of a warm up is not to push yourself to exhaustion. You just want to get "warmed up".

After 3 minutes, increase the speed a little bit to make it a little more challenging and really get your heart pumping harder. Maintain this speed for another 4 minutes.

Then, increase the speed another level and maintain that for the final 3 minutes.

Beginner Butt Lifting and Shaping Workout #1 (No Equipment)

Perform each of these exercises for 30 seconds. Repeat the full series 6 times for a total of 15 minutes.

1. **Basic Squats**

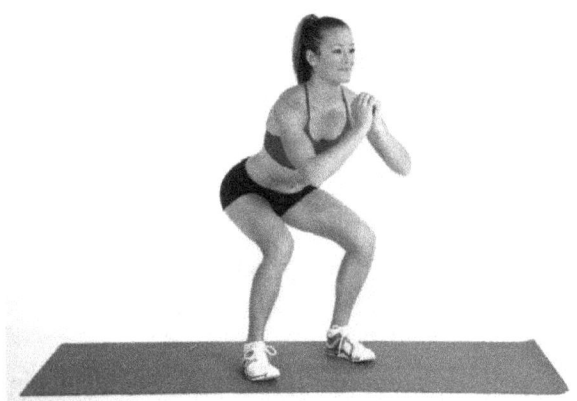

Start in a standing position with your feet standing wider than hip width apart. They should be 12" to 18" inches apart. Place your hands on your hips and then bend your knees to get into a squat position. Hold this for 30 seconds.

2. **Bridge Lifts**

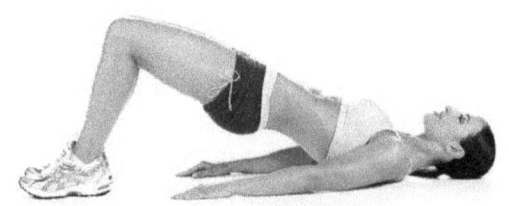

Lie down on your back with your knees bent and feet flat on the floor. Your feet should be placed just wider than hip width apart.

Your arms should be straight at your sides with palms on the floor. From this position, pull your pelvis upward toward the ceiling.

Let the power come entirely from your thighs. Push upward until only your feet and shoulders (and arms) are touching the floor.

Lower yourself back down. Continue lifting and lowering for 30 seconds.

3. *Chair Pose with Leg Extensions*

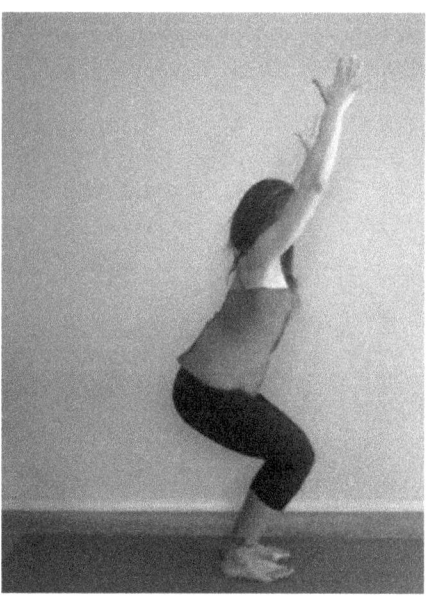

Start in a standing position with your legs hip width apart. Bend your knees and lean your torso forward slightly.

You should look as if you are just about to sit down in a chair. While in this position, kick your right leg up in front of you as high as you can while maintaining balance and keeping your right leg straight.

Lower it back down. Do the same move with your left leg.

Remain in chair pose and continue alternating between extending your right and left legs for 30 seconds.

4. *Plank with Leg Lifts*

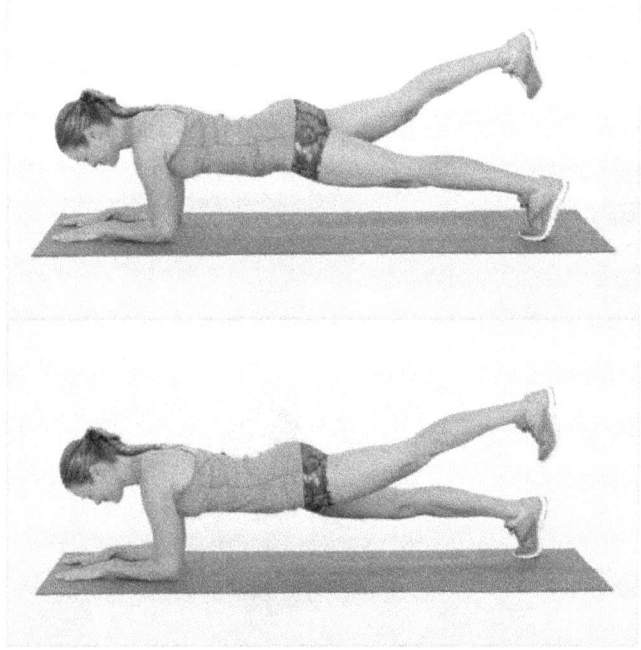

Lie down on your stomach. Lift your upper body up and rest on your elbows with your palms on the floor and your elbows forming 90° angles.

Push onto your toes and then lift up into plank position. While in this position, lift your right leg up toward the ceiling as high as you can while keeping it straight.

Lower your leg back down. Do the same move with your left leg. Continue alternating between each leg for 30 seconds.

5. *Reverse Lunges*

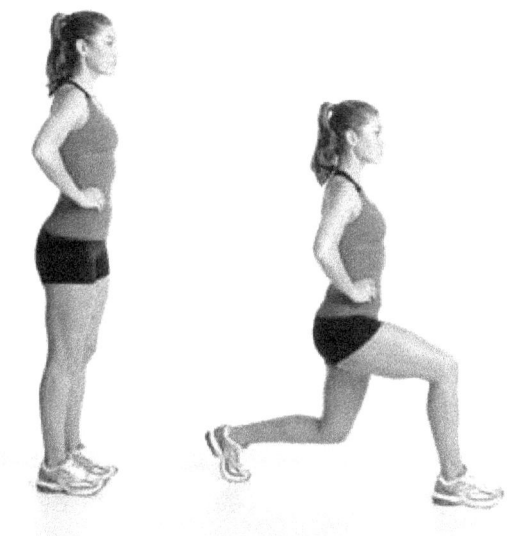

Start in a standing position with your legs hip width apart. Kick your right leg back into a lunge.

Push your pelvis toward the floor and really feel the stretch of the lunge. Then lift your right leg up and come back to a standing position.

Kick your left leg back into a lunge, really push deep into the lunge and feel the stretch. Return to standing. Continue alternating between your right and left legs for 30 seconds.

Beginner Butt Lifting and Shaping Workout #2 (With Equipment)

Perform each of the 5 exercises for 30 seconds. Repeat the full series 6 times for a total of 15 minutes.

Equipment Needed: Resistance Band

1. Bridge Lifts with Resistance Band

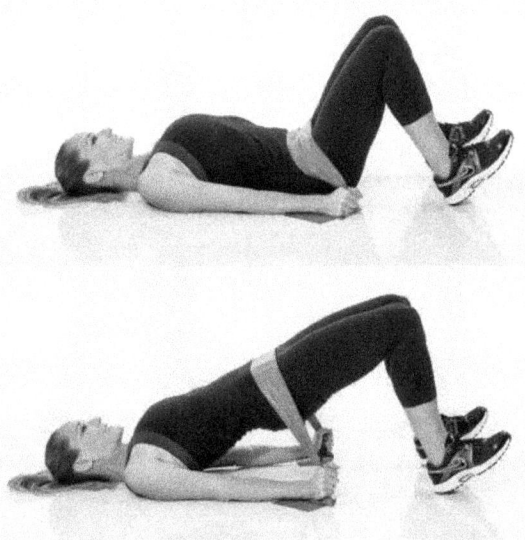

Lie on your back with your knees bent and your feet planted firmly on the floor. Hold a resistance band across your stomach and make sure that you are pulling it tightly toward the floor.

Lift your butt and pelvis off the floor and push them high up toward the ceiling until only your arms, shoulders, and feet are touching the floor. Lower yourself back down. Continue lifting and lowering yourself for 30 seconds.

Make sure that the resistance band is providing enough pressure to make the lifts more challenging.

2. **Bridge Pose with Leg Lifts using Resistance Band**

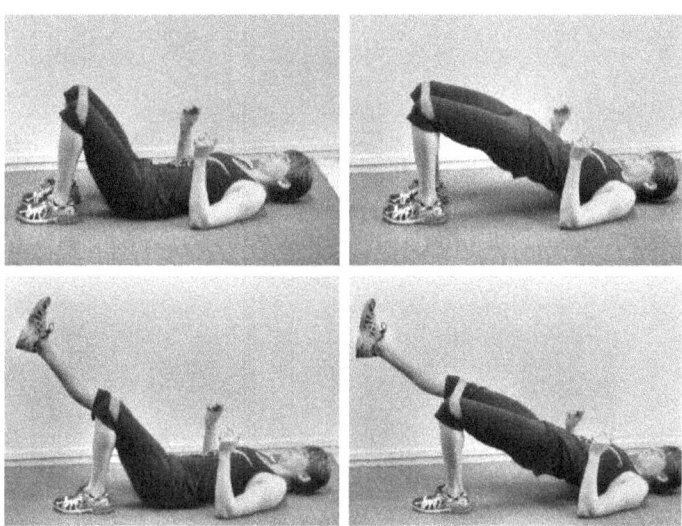

Return to bridge pose with your body lifted off the floor. This time, you should have the resistance band tied securely around your thighs.

While in bridge pose, push your right thigh up and toward your stomach as far as you can. Be careful to maintain balance with your left leg.

Lower your leg back down. Repeat the move with your left leg. Continue doing leg lifts with alternating legs for 30 seconds.

3. **Leg Raises with Resistance Band**

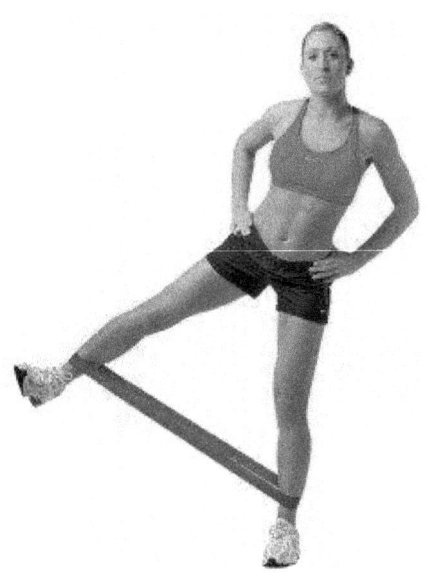

Stand up with your legs hip width apart and the resistance band tied securely around your calves.

Kick your right leg back and up as far as you can while keeping the leg straight. Return it back to the floor. Repeat the move with your left leg.

Continue doing leg raises with alternating legs for 30 seconds.

4. *Squats with Side Leg Lifts using Resistance Band*

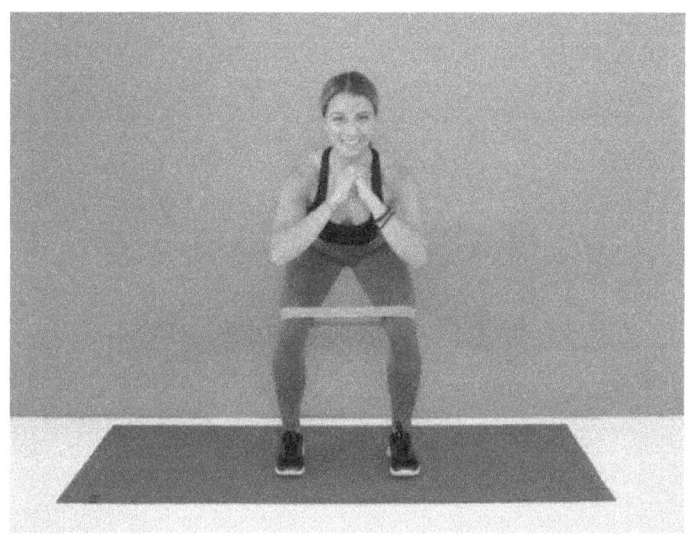

Stand with your feet about 12" to 18" apart. Make sure the resistance band is tied securely around your calves. You should already feel some pressure or resistance from it with your legs spread this far.

Bend at your knees to go into a squat position. Keep your hands on your hips. Kick your right leg up and out to the side while balancing on your left leg.

Go as far as you can without changing the position of your leg. Bring your foot back to the floor.

Do the same thing with your left leg. Remain in the squat position doing side lifts with alternating legs for 30 seconds.

5. *Reclined Hamstring Curls with Resistance Band*

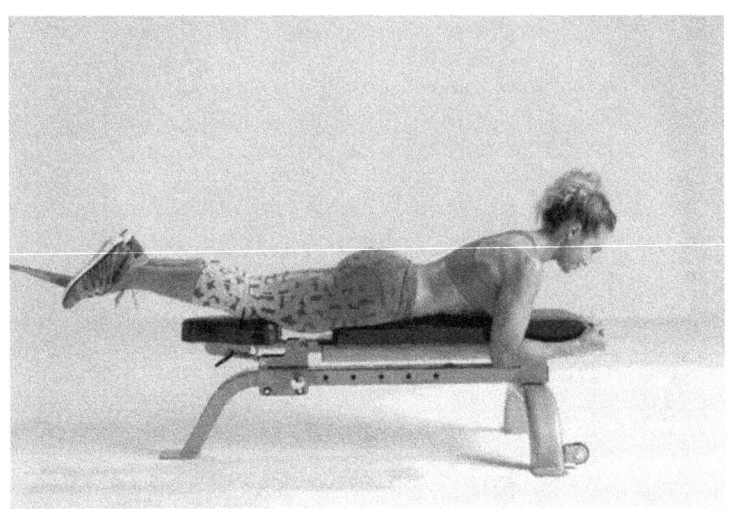

Tie your resistance band to bed posts or other sturdy anchoring points.

Lie down on your stomach. Bend your legs up and slip the resistance band around your calves.

Pull your feet (and the resistance band) down toward your butt as far as you can. Release your legs back up. Continue this for 30 seconds.

Beginner Butt Lifting and Shaping Workout #3 (Cardio Based)

Option 1:

Stair Climbing

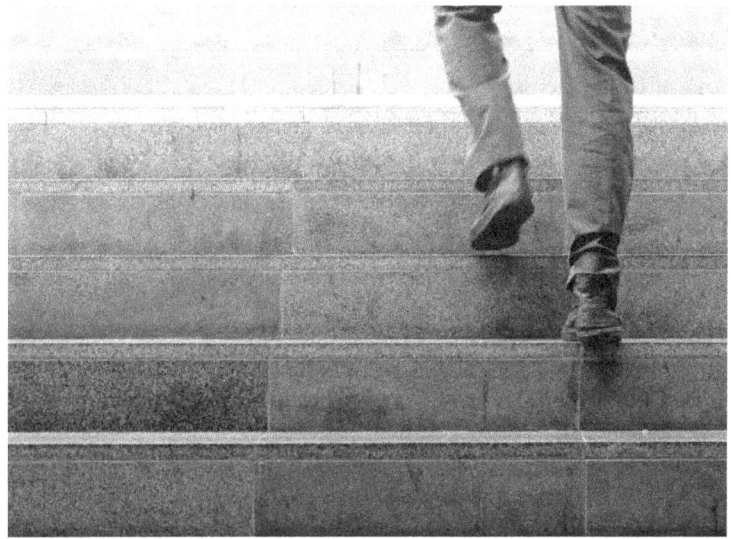

Use a stair climbing machine or a fairly tall set of stairs. Climb up the stairs, one or two steps at a time, at your maximum speed (but not so fast that you trip and fall) for 20 seconds.

Then climb up the stairs at a more moderate speed for 40 seconds. Continue alternating between these intervals for 15 minutes.

As you improve, increase the length of your high intensity interval and decrease the length of your low intensity interval until you are able to do 40 seconds of high intensity and 20 seconds of low intensity.

Option 2:

Hiking or Mountain Climbing

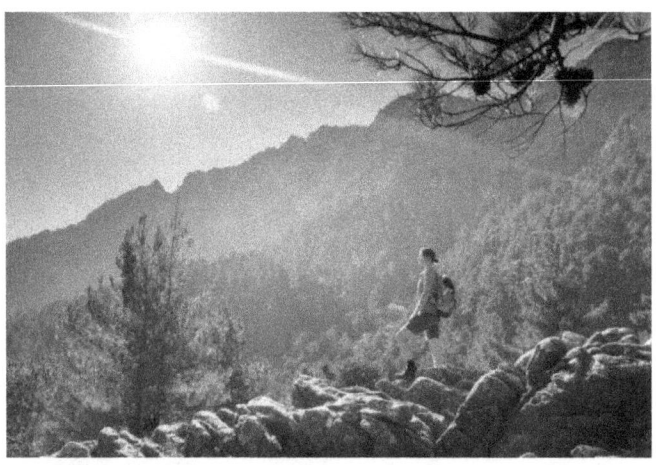

If you have mountains or large hills nearby, go out hiking or mountain climbing in order to meet your workout requirements.

Incorporate intervals by hiking at your maximum speed for 20 seconds and then hiking at a more moderate speed for 40 seconds.

Continue these intervals for at least 15 minutes (you can of course go for longer if you like).

Slowly increase your high intensity intervals and decrease your low intensity intervals as your fitness improves until you reach 40 seconds of high intensity and 20 seconds of low intensity.

10 Minute Cool Down

Your cool down should start with a light cardio (even lower intensity than your warm up was). You need to transition your body out of workout mode and back into its regular speed.

So, walk, skip rope, or do any other cardio activity that you enjoy. We'll use skipping rope again as we did in the warm up.

Skip rope for 5 minutes at the same speed that you started your warm up with.

After 5 minutes, you need to stretch. Start in a standing position. Step your right leg back into a deep lunge.

Drop your right knee to the floor and let your shin and the top of your foot rest on the floor.

Hold this for 30 seconds. Then slowly drop your left knee to the side and let your front calf rest on the floor. Your front calf should be perpendicular to your right leg.

Put your palms on the floor just in front of your calf and lean forward. You will feel the stretch along the top of your right thigh and along the inside of your left thigh. Hold this for 30 seconds. Lift back out of it and then lunge with your left leg back this time.

Hold that lunge for 30 seconds before moving again into this second stretch with your left leg forward and calf resting sideways on the floor.

Lay back on your back with your toes pointed toward the wall furthest from you. Bring your right knee up.

Clasp your hands around your shin and pull it into your chest. Hold for 30 seconds. Repeat this with your left leg. Release and put both legs on the floor.

Lift your right knee up again but this time cross it over to the side and let it drop to the floor on the outside of your left thigh. Your right foot should be in line with your left knee.

Keep your back flat against the floor. Place your left hand on your right knee and push your knee toward the floor. Hold this for 30 seconds. Repeat it again with your other leg.

15-Minute Advanced Butt Workouts

If the beginner workouts are too easy for you, kick it up a notch with the workouts in these chapters to make sure your butt is getting the full advantages of your daily 15 minutes of butt firming exercise!

10 Minute Warm Up

The perfect warm up for your butt lifting and shaping workout is some stair climbing. If you've got stairs in your house, these will work perfectly.

If not, find some stairs or a steep hill outside that you can use.

Go up and down the steps, one step at a time, at a moderate pace for 3 minutes.

After that first 3 minutes is up, go at a slightly faster pace and climb the stairs 2 steps at a time.

Do this for 3 minutes. Then, go back down to the bottom and jump up onto the first step. Then jump back down to the floor.

Repeat this for 2 minutes. For the final 2 minutes of the warm up, climb the stairs 2 steps at a time at the pace you were going before the stair jumping.

Advanced Butt Lifting and Shaping Workout #1 (No Equipment)

Do each exercise for 60 seconds and then repeat the series 3 times for a total of 15 minutes.

1. *Bow Pose*

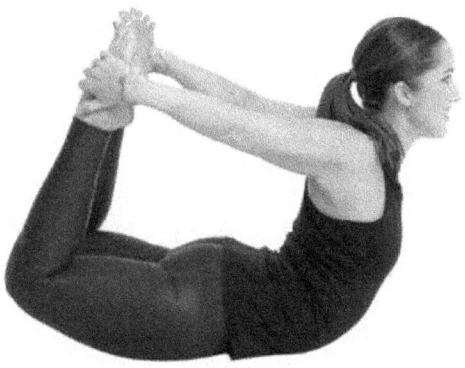

Lie down flat on your stomach. Bend your knees and touch your heels to your butt. Reach back with both arms and grab each ankle.

Now, lift your chest and thighs off the floor at the same time. Push your ankles up and away from your body.

When you are fully in this pose, the only part of you that will be touching the floor is your lower abdomen.

Hold this pose for 60 seconds.

2. Plank to Forward Bend

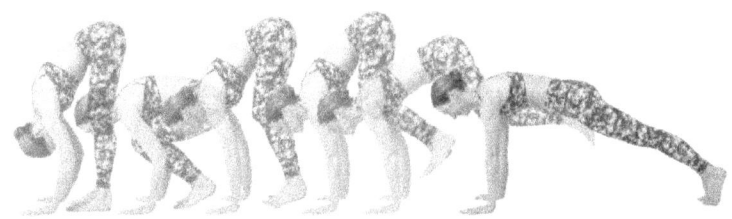

Begin by lying on your stomach. Lift your upper body up and rest on your elbows. Your arms should be parallel with each other.

Your palms should be flat on the floor and your elbows should be bent to form a 90° angle. Bend your feet so that your toes are pressed into the floor.

Lift yourself up into a plank position. From this position jump your legs up and in to move into a forward bend.

The forward bend is when your feet are together, your legs are straight, and your torso is bent all the way forward so that your palms are touching the floor.

Once you have jumped into a forward bend, jump back into plank position. At no point should your palms leave the floor.

Continue jumping between plank pose and forward bend as fast as you can for 60 seconds.

3. Frog Pose

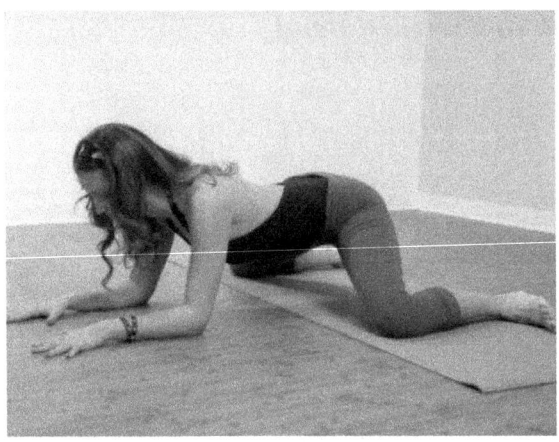

Lay back down on your stomach with your toes pointed and the tops of your feet flat on the floor. Bend your right leg so that your foot touches your butt.

Lift your upper torso up so that your arms are straight and your palms are on the floor supporting your weight.

Lift up as high as you can so that your butt and back meet at a 90°-degree angle (or as close to that as you can).

Bring your right hand on top of your right foot and push it down as far as you can. You will feel the stretch in the front of your thigh.

But it is also shaping your butt and deepening that crease that separates the bottom of your butt from your upper thigh. Hold this for 30 seconds then release and do the same thing with your left leg.

4. *Upward Bow Pose*

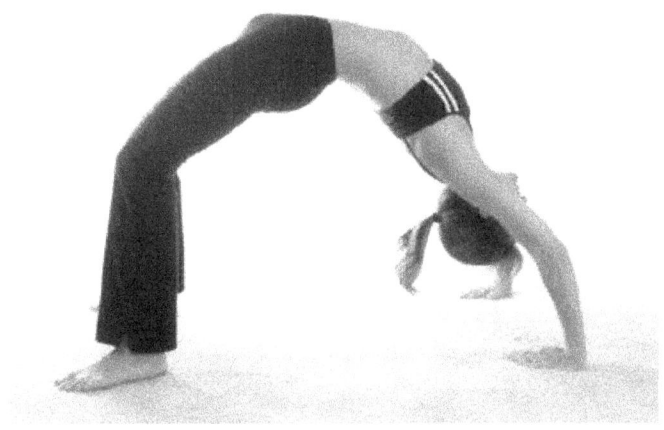

Lie down on your back this time. Bend your knees and put your feet flat against the floor. Your legs should be spread slightly wider than hip width apart.

With your palms facing the floor, reach your arms up above your head. Bend your hands back and place your palms on the floor just above your head.

Use your thighs to press up and lift your entire body (including head) off the floor. Your head will hang and look at the wall behind you.

Pretend there is a string tied to your belly button that is drawing it up toward the ceiling. Flex your thighs and let the power come from this area.

Hold the pose for 60 seconds. (Take rests if you need to, this pose can be challenging).

When you come back down, start by slowly lowering your head to the floor, then your shoulders, then your upper back, lower back, and finally your butt.

5. *Camel Pose to Child Pose*

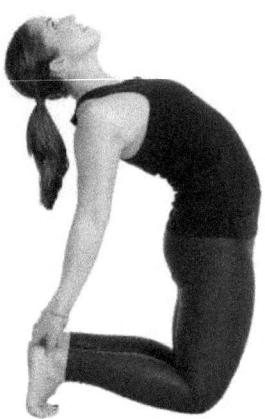

Kneel down onto your knees with your shins and the tops of your feet flat against the floor. Draw your upper body and thighs up so that your knees form a 90° angle.

Reach back and clasp each of your ankles. Bend your upper body back into this pose so that you can look at the wall behind you. Once in position, lift out, drop your thighs onto your calves and lean your torso forward to put your forehead on the ground.

This is child pose. Continue rapidly moving between these 2 poses for the full 60 seconds.

Advanced Butt Lifting and Shaping Workout #2 (With Equipment)

Equipment Needed: Resistance Band, Ankle Weights

Do each exercise for 60 seconds and then repeat the series 3 times for a total of 15 minutes.

1. ***Reverse Leg Lift with Resistance Band and Ankle Weights***

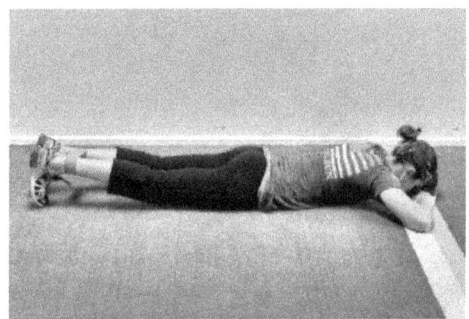

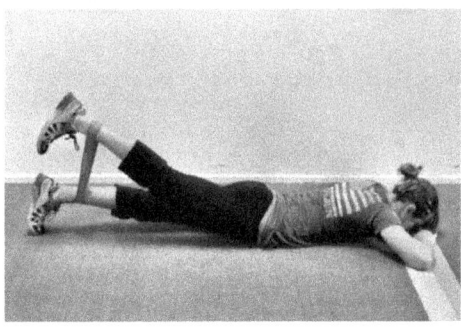

Lie down on your stomach with your legs straight out behind you.

You should have ankle weights on and a resistance band tied tightly around your thighs just above your knees. Bend your right knee up so that your foot is pointing at the ceiling.

Now, lift your right thigh up as far as you can, feeling the resistance of the band tied around you. Continue to lift your thigh up and down without letting your knee touch the floor for 30 seconds.

Then repeat this exercise with your left leg.

2. *Squats with Resistance Band and Ankle Weights*

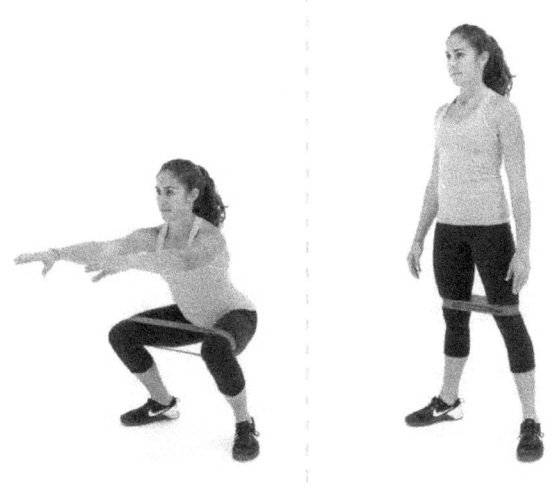

Keep your ankle weights on but move the resistance band so that it is tied tightly around your calves. Start in a standing position with your legs hip width apart.

Push your right leg out to the side as far as you can with the resistance band and then push down into a deep squat. Stand back up and move your right leg in. Then, do the same thing with your left leg.

Continue alternating between your left and right leg (remembering to always do a deep squat after you step out) as rapidly as you can for the full 60 seconds.

3. *Stair Climbing with Resistance Band and Ankle Weights*

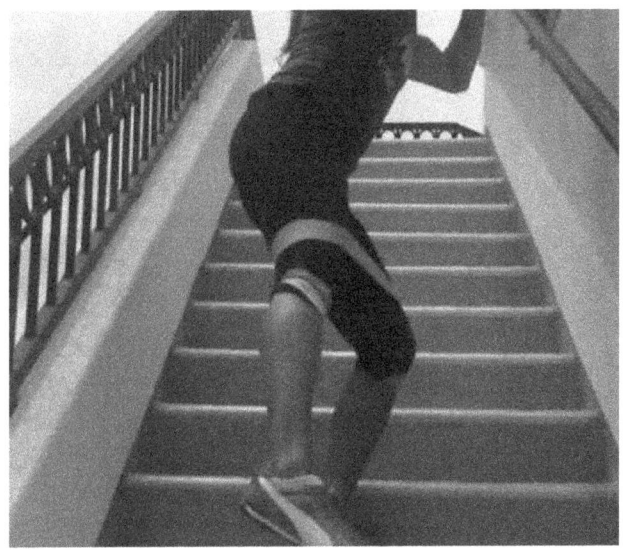

Tie the resistance band around your thighs just above your knees. The ankle weights should also be on.

Climb stairs one step at a time as quickly as you can (but maintain a speed slow enough that you can still focus on balance and form).

The resistance band and ankle weights will add even more intensity to a stair climbing routine. Continue climbing for 60 seconds.

4. *Reclined Hamstring Curl with Resistance Band and Ankle Weights*

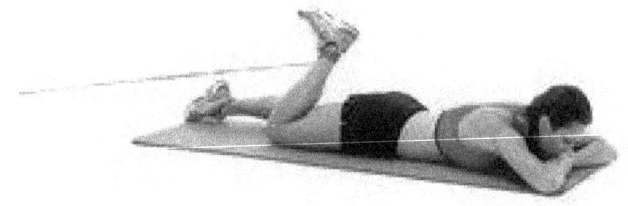

Tie your resistance band to bedposts or other sturdy anchoring points in your house. Make sure your ankle weights are in place.

Lay down on your stomach and slip the band around your calves. Pull your feet (and the resistance band) toward your butt.

Lift your legs back up. Repeat this for the full 60 seconds.

5. *Forward Bend with Leg Lifts using Resistance Band and Ankle Weights*

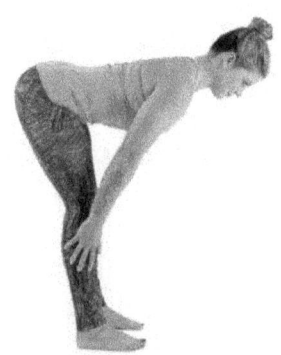

Stand up straight with your ankle weights on and your resistance band tied snuggly around your calves. Bend your torso forward to put your palms on the floor. Keep your knees straight.

If you can't touch the floor while keeping your knees straight, just go as far down as you can. Once in a forward bend, lift your right leg back behind you as high as you can (while keeping it straight).

Bring it back down. Do the same move with your left leg. Continue alternating between your left and right leg for 60 seconds.

Advanced Butt Lifting and Shaping Workout #3 (Cardio Based)

Option 1:

Stair Climbing

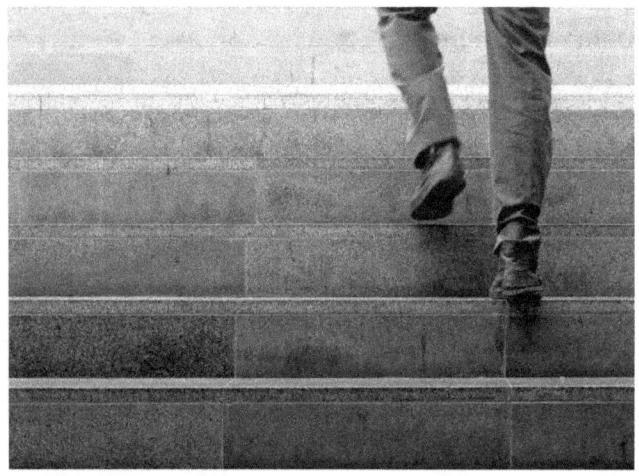

Climbing upstairs is one of the greatest exercises you can do to give your butt the absolute perfect shape. It's actually great for your legs as well but you'll see the most impressive benefits in your butt.

The incline causes your body to draw the most power from your upper thighs, butt, hips, and lower back in order to lift itself.

You can either use a stair climber machine or find a nice tall set of stairs outside. If neither of those is an option, stairs in your house will work just fine.

To start this workout, run up the stairs one or two steps at a time as fast as you possibly can (without falling!) for 40 seconds.

Ideally, the stairs you are using should be tall enough that you can run at maximum speed for 40 seconds without reaching the top. After that 40 seconds, continue climbing at a more moderate speed for 20 seconds.

If you reach the top at any point during these intervals, just go back down and start again. Continue alternating between these intervals for 15 minutes.

Option 2:

Hiking or Mountain Climbing

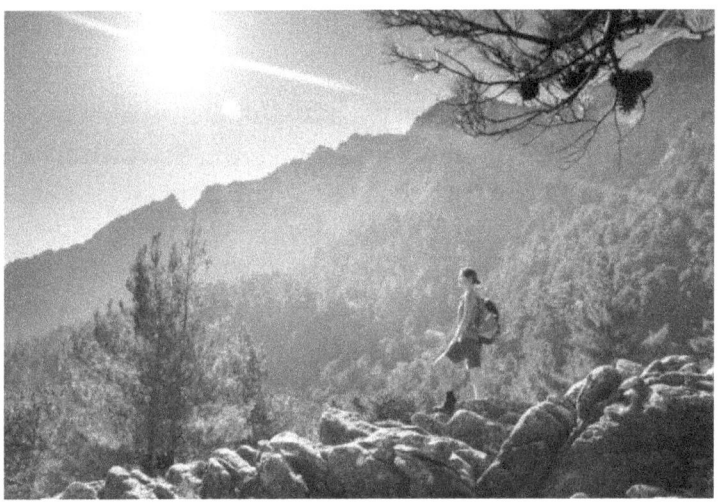

If you prefer to get out into the great outdoors and you live within reasonable distance of a mountain or particularly large hill, then hiking or mountain climbing can be a great addition to your weekly workout schedule to keep things interesting.

If hiking, start with 40 seconds of running at maximum speed and then slow down to a more moderate hiking speed for 20 seconds.

Continue to alternate between these high intensity and low intensity intervals for a total of 15 minutes.

While mountain climbing, you'll probably have less opportunity to safely go at high speeds while scaling a cliff.

However, mountain climbing is a great workout that combines cardio and strength training into one (and also happens to be super fun and exciting!) so just take it at a safe speed but do go as quickly as you can without sacrificing skill and agility.

Spend at least 15 minutes climbing upward.

10 Minute Cool Down

After any of these high intensity butt-shaping workouts, you are going to need to take 10 minutes to cool down. Start with 5 minutes of light cardio. You can jog in place, do jumping jacks, skip with a jump rope, take a walk around the block, or anything else that gets you moving at a moderate pace.

After 5 minutes of light cardio, do some stretches. Your thighs and glutes got the most of your butt workout so you want to target those areas for your stretches.

Start with some deep lunges. From a standing position, step your right leg straight behind you and get into a lunge.

Let your knee rest on the floor and flatten your foot so that the top of it is also resting on the floor. Lean forward on your front thigh and feel the deep stretch on your inner thighs. Hold this for 60 seconds. Repeat this with the other leg forward.

Sit down on the floor with your legs straight out in front of you. Bend your right knee up. Step your right foot across to the outer side of your left thigh. Use your left arm to hug your knee into your chest.

Twist your upper body to look over to the right and place your right hand, palm side down, on the floor behind you.

You should feel the stretch in your outer thigh and along your right side. Hold this for 60 seconds. Repeat the same thing with your left leg.

Lay down on your back with your knees bent and your feet flat on the floor. Cross your right leg so that your right foot is resting against your left knee (similar to a cross legged sitting position but while laying down).

Pull your left leg up and clasp your hands around your left thigh.

Pull it in toward your chest as far as you can. You will feel the stretch along the back of your right thigh. Hold this for 30 seconds. Repeat the same thing with your left leg.

I hope you have learned something from this book so far and would greatly appreciate it if you could leave an honest review on Amazon.com.

15-Minute Beginner Leg Workouts

With your back and butt worked, it's time to move all the way down to your legs. In this chapter, you'll get 3 great 15-minute workouts that are perfect for beginners.

10 Minute Warm Up

For this warm up, you'll want to make sure your legs take on most of the work so that they are warmed and ready when you start one of the following workouts.

Get on the treadmill or go out for a walk. Start at a moderate speed. It should be faster than your regular walking speed but far from a jogging or running speed. Walk at this speed for 3 minutes.

After that, increase the speed to the fastest speed you can walk without breaking into a jog. Maintain that speed for 3 minutes. Now, increase the speed so that you are in a light jog. Maintain this speed for 4 minutes.

You can also do a variation of this on a stationary bike or road bike. Start cycling at a moderate pace for 3 minutes. Increase it slightly for the next 3 minutes. Then bump the intensity enough to break a sweat without getting exhausted for the final 4 minutes.

Beginner Leg Carving and Toning Workout #1 (No Equipment)

For this workout, you will do each exercise for 30 seconds at a time and then repeat the series 6 times.

1. **Chair Pose**

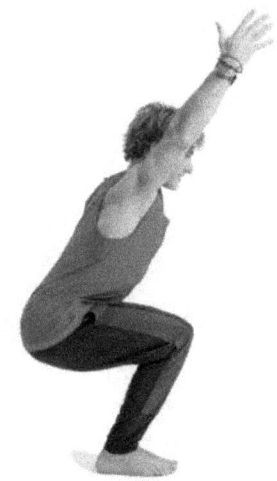

Start in a standing position with your legs hip width apart.

Bend at the knees and lean your torso forward slightly so that you look as if you are just about to sit down in a chair. Hold this position for 30 seconds without moving.

2. **Calf Raises**

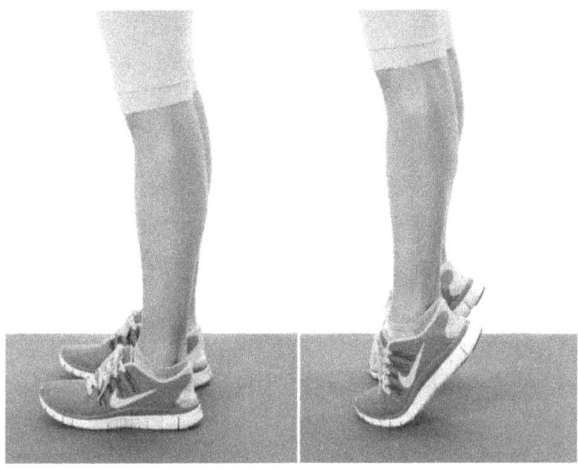

Find a stair or a ledge. Stand at the edge so that only the balls of your feet and your toes are on the edge. Your heels should be hanging off.

Raise your heels up as high as you can. Hold this position for one breath. Lower your heels down as far as you can without falling off. Hold this position for one breath. Repeat this for the full 30 seconds.

3. *Squats to Wide Legged Stretch*

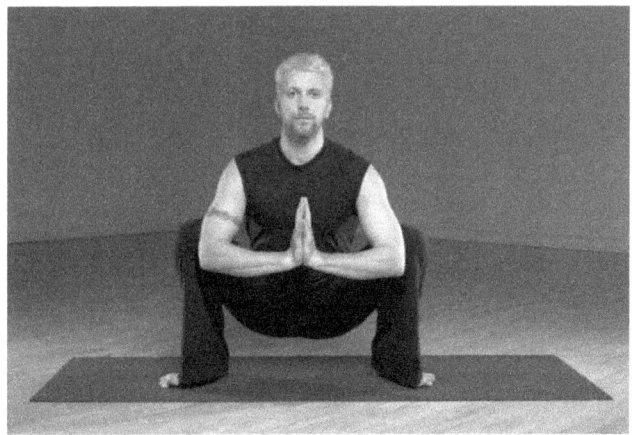

Start with your legs spread as far apart as you can get them while maintaining your balance. Bend down at the knees into a squat position.

Hold this for 5 seconds. Then, straighten your knees again. As you straighten your knees, bend your torso forward at the hips and put your palms on the floor.

With your legs straight, touch your head to the floor. If you can't touch your head to the floor, that's ok.

Just go as low as you can while keeping your legs straight. Hold this for 2 seconds. Lift your torso up halfway so that it is parallel to the floor. Bend your knees back into a squat position.

Repeat this cycle for the full 30 seconds.

4. *Squats with Side Steps*

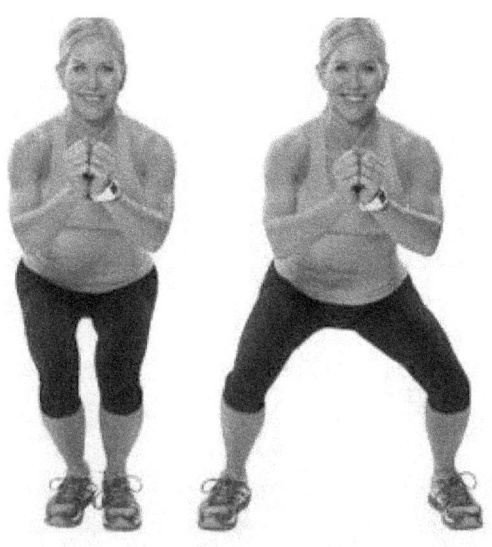

Get into a squat position again. This time, however, your legs should be a little less far apart.

While staying in this squat position, lift your right leg up and take a step to the right side. Then, lift your left leg up and take a step to the left side.

Continue stepping from side to side without ever lifting out of the squat position. Continue this for the full 30 seconds.

5. *Half Moon Pose*

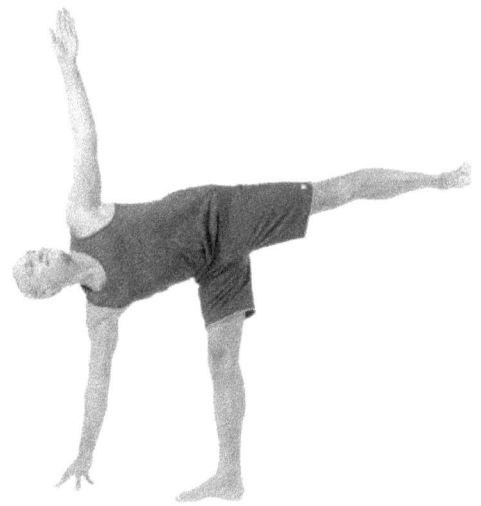

Stand with your legs hip width apart. Reach your arms up above you. Slowly bend your torso at your hips while lifting your right leg out behind you at the same time.

Lower your left arm down to the floor but don't place any weight on it. Just use this arm to help maintain balance. All the weight should be on your left leg.

Your right leg should be straight out behind you so that it is parallel with the floor. Your torso should also be parallel with the floor. Your arms should form a straight vertical line between the ground and ceiling.

Hold this for 30 seconds. Each time you come to this exercise, use a different leg so that each leg has done the exercise 3 times by the time your 15 minutes is up.

Beginner Leg Carving and Toning Workout #2 (With Equipment)

Equipment Needed: Resistance Band and Ankle Weights

Do each exercise for 30 seconds and then repeat the series. You'll repeat the series 6 times for a total of 15 minutes.

1. *Reclined Leg Lifts with Ankle Weights*

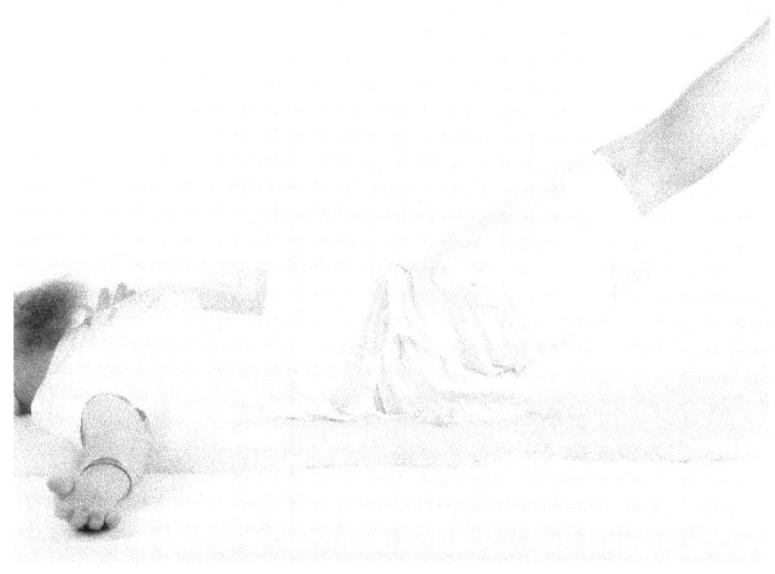

Start by lying down on your back with your legs straight. You should have ankle weights wrapped around your ankles. Point your toes out so that your feet are parallel with the floor.

Lift your legs up together without bending your knees. Lift them to a 45°-degree angle. Then lower them down to the floor. Repeat this for 30 seconds.

2. Reclined Corkscrew with Ankle Weights

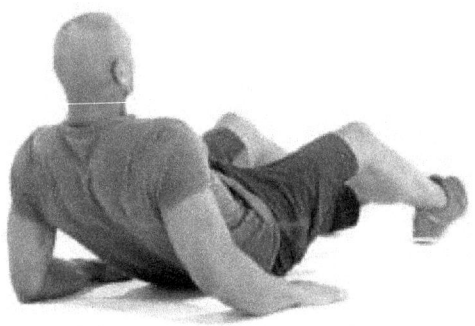

Again, you will be lying on the floor with your ankle weights wrapped around your ankles. Point your toes and lift your legs straight up so that they are perpendicular with the ground. Lower them to the side until they form a 45° angle with the floor.

Then, circle them around to the center and then to your other side. Then lift them back up. Always try to maintain that 45° angle with the floor. Do this as one continuous motion for the full 30 seconds.

3. Air Cycling with Ankle Weights

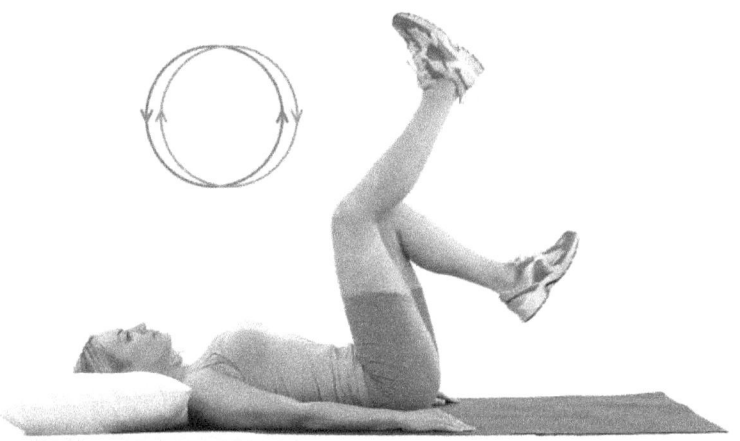

Continue to lie down. With your ankle weights still attached, raise your legs above your as you did in the last exercise. This time, lift your butt a few inches off the floor.

Your arms should be straight at your sides with palms facing the floor. Use your arms to maintain balance while your butt is raised.

Now, start to bend your legs in a cycling motion (as if you were on a bicycle). Make sure your butt doesn't touch the floor at any point. Do this for a full 30 seconds.

4. *Standing with One Leg Raised using Resistance Band*

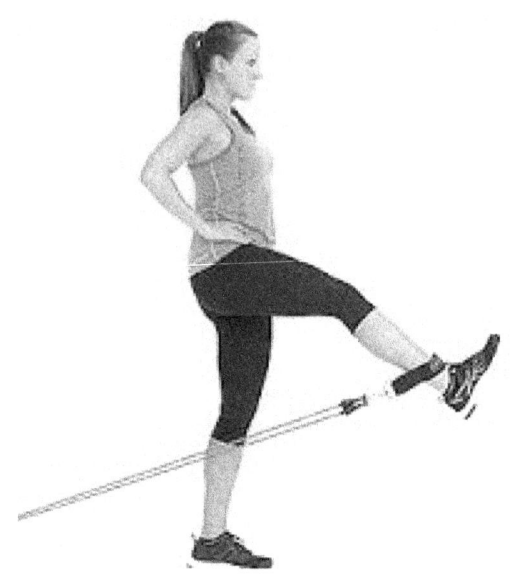

For this exercise, you should remove your ankle weights. If you feel confident, you can leave them on. Stand with your legs hip width apart.

Bend your right knee up and wrap your resistance band around the bottom of your foot. Push your right leg forward and out so that it is straight in front of you. Push your foot against the resistance band and make sure to keep your knee completely straight.

Hold this pose for the full 30 seconds. Each time you do this exercise, alternate legs so that by the end of the 15 minutes, each leg has been raised and stretched 3 times.

5. *Reclined Leg Lifts (reverse side) with Ankle Weights*

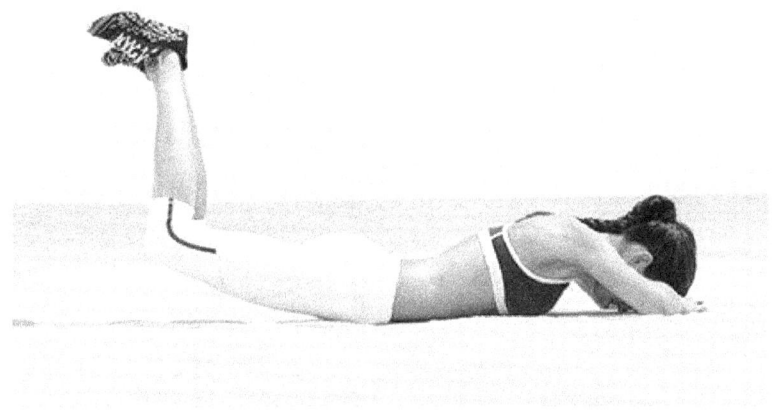

Put your ankle weights back on for this exercise. Lay down flat on your stomach with your legs straight.

Bend your knees and lift your legs up and toward your butt. Then lower them down to the floor again. Repeat this for 30 seconds.

Beginner Leg Carving and Toning Workout #3 (Cardio Based)

Option 1:

Swimming

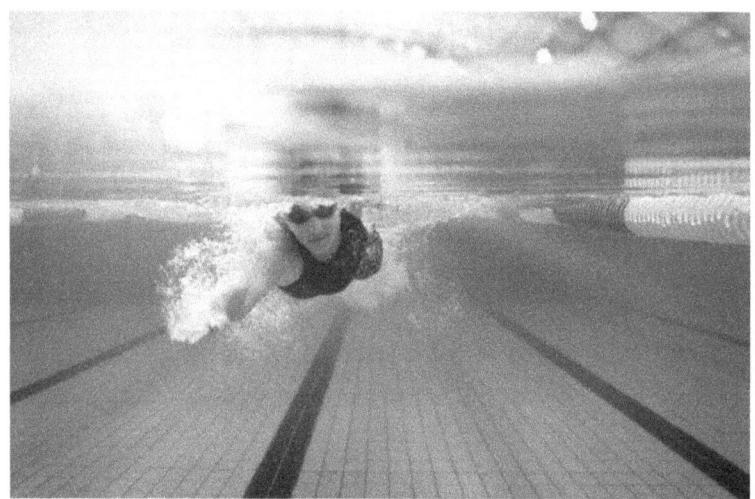

Swimming is a great workout for your whole body but most of the power comes from your legs. If you have your own pool, that's perfect.

If not, many gyms have a pool onsite. Often, it's even an indoor pool which means you can even do this work out during the winter months.

After doing your warm up, get in the pool and swim laps. Swim at your maximum speed for 20 seconds. Then, swim at a more moderate speed for 40 seconds.

You will probably just have to count off the seconds in your head as you won't be able to hear any timer while underwater. Continue alternating between high intensity and low intensity swimming for 15 minutes.

If you don't have a clock nearby, that means you will do 15 20-second intervals of high intensity swimming and 15 40-second intervals of low intensity swimming.

As you improve, change the intervals to 25 seconds of high intensity and 35 seconds of low intensity. Then, change it to 30 seconds of high intensity and 30 seconds of low intensity.

Your goal is to eventually reach 40 seconds of high intensity and 20 seconds of low intensity.

Option 2:

Cycling (Stationary or Outdoor)

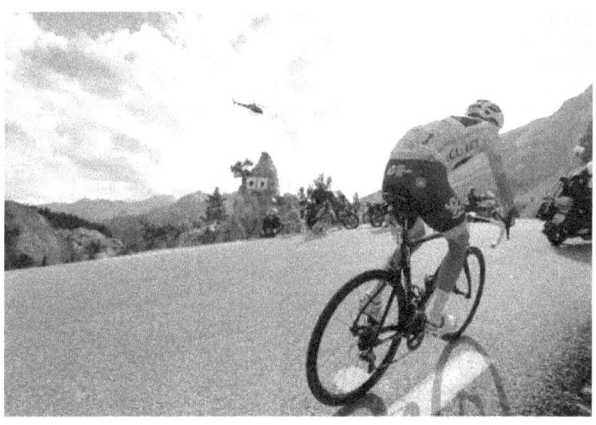

If you aren't a fan of swimming or getting access to a pool is just not a realistic option for you, cycling is also a great cardio workout for the legs.

You can either get a stationary bike to use at home or use a road bike to cycle outdoors. Just as with the swimming, you'll do high intensity and low intensity intervals.

Start with 20 seconds of cycling at your maximum speed. If you have a stationary bike with options to change the settings, you should also increase the resistance during these 20 seconds.

If you are cycling outdoors, shift to the higher gears to increase the resistance. Cycle as fast as you can at this increased resistance for 20 seconds.

After the 20 seconds is up, switch to a lower gear or decrease the resistance setting on your stationary bike and cycle at a moderate speed for 40 seconds.

Continue alternating between these high intensity and low intensity intervals for 15 minutes. Increase the length of your high intensity interval and decrease the length of your low intensity interval as you start to improve.

Again, your goal is to eventually reach 40 seconds of high intensity cycling and 20 seconds of low intensity cycling.

10 Minute Cool Down

To cool down after any of these 3 workouts, you want to make sure your legs get a good stretch so that the muscles stay flexible. Start with some light cardio.

This can be moderate walking, cycling, or swimming for 5 minutes. Don't strain yourself. Just keep your legs moving so that they can gradually transition out of workout mode.

After 5 minutes of walking, move on to the stretching. Lay down on your back. Point your toes forward. Bend your right knee into your chest. Wrap your resistance band around the bottom of your foot and then stretch your leg up above until your knee is straight.

Use the resistance band to pull your leg down toward your head but always keep your knee straight.

Pull on the resistance band enough so that you can feel the stretch through the back of your leg. Hold for 30 seconds. Repeat this again with the other leg.

Continue to lie down. Keep your toes pointed. Bend your right leg into your chest again. This time, clasp your hands around your shin and pull the leg deep into your chest. Hold this for 30 seconds. Repeat it again with the other leg.

Sit up and open your legs as wide as you can. Use your hands to pull them a little wider. Make sure your knees stay straight. Bend to your right side.

Reach your left arm up over your head and clasp your toes. If you can't reach your toes, that's okay. Just go as far as you can. Hold that stretch for 30 seconds. Repeat this again on the other side.

Keep your legs open. This time bend straight forward between your legs and touch your head to the floor (or as close to the floor as you can get).

Reach your arms out in front of you and rest your palms on the floor. Feel the stretch in your inner thighs. Hold this for 30 seconds. Bend your legs in so that the soles of your feet are touching.

Clasp your hands on your shins and pull your feet closer in toward your pelvis. Push your knees toward the floor and bend forward.

Continue to push your knees as close to the floor as you can get them. Hold this pose for 30 seconds.

Lay down on your stomach. Bend your right leg in toward your butt. Clasp your ankle. Use your hand to pull your leg up toward your head until you feel a good stretch along the front of your thigh. Hold this for 30 seconds. Repeat it again with the left leg.

15-Minute Advanced Leg Workouts

This chapter contains the last set of workouts. Like the previous chapter, it focuses on leg strengthening. If you feel the beginner workouts from the previous chapter are too easy and want to move on immediately to these, proceed with caution.

The second workout uses a pull up bar. Don't strain yourself with this one as you could cause serious damage if you overdo it.

Test out your abilities by doing a modified, shorter version of the workout (try 7.5 minutes instead of the full 15). Again, always remember to do your warm up before and your cool down after!

10 Minute Warm Up

For your warm up, hop on a treadmill or go outside. Start walking at a moderate speed. After 2 minutes, increase the speed a little bit.

After another 2 minutes at the speed, increase the speed again until you are in a light jog. Maintain this speed for 3 minutes. Increase the speed again so that you are in a more intense jog (but still nowhere near your maximum speed).

Maintain that speed for 3 minutes.

Now you are ready to start one of the following workouts.

Advanced Leg Carving and Toning Workout #1 (No Equipment)

Set a time and do each exercise for 60 seconds. Cycle through the series 3 times.

1. **Frog Leaps**

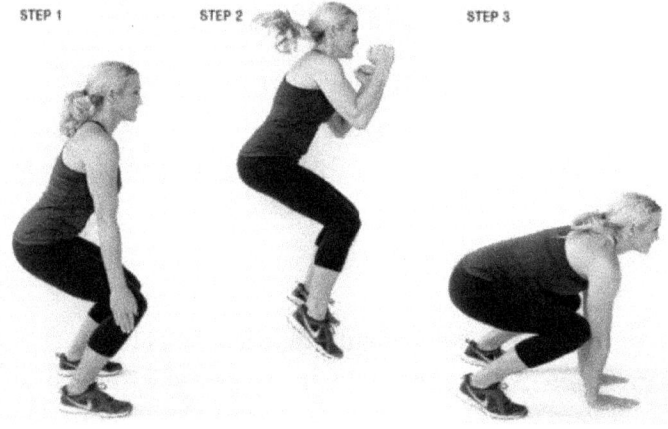

Start with your legs hip width apart. Crouch down so that you are balancing on your toes with your knees bent and your palms are flat against the floor between your legs.

From this position, leap straight up into the air. Raise your arms up as you are jumping up.

When your toes touch the floor again, immediately crouch back down into your frog pose.

2. **Lunges with Knee Drops**

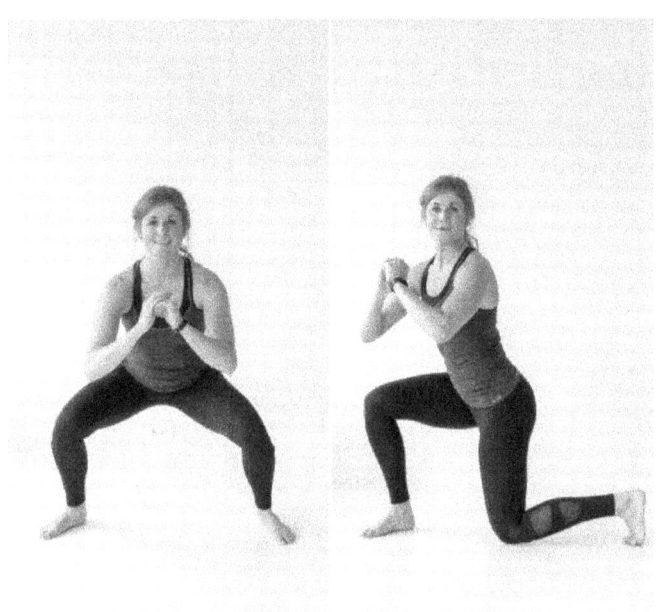

Start in a standing position, legs hip width apart. Draw your left leg behind you into a deep lunge. Your back leg should be straight and your front leg should be bent into a 90° angle.

Drop your back knee down to touch the floor (but don't actually put any weight on your knee). Raise it back up to a straight position.

Continue dropping and raising your knee. Halfway through (30 seconds), switch legs so that your right leg is now the back leg. Repeat the knee drops with this leg.

3. *Plank with Side Jumps*

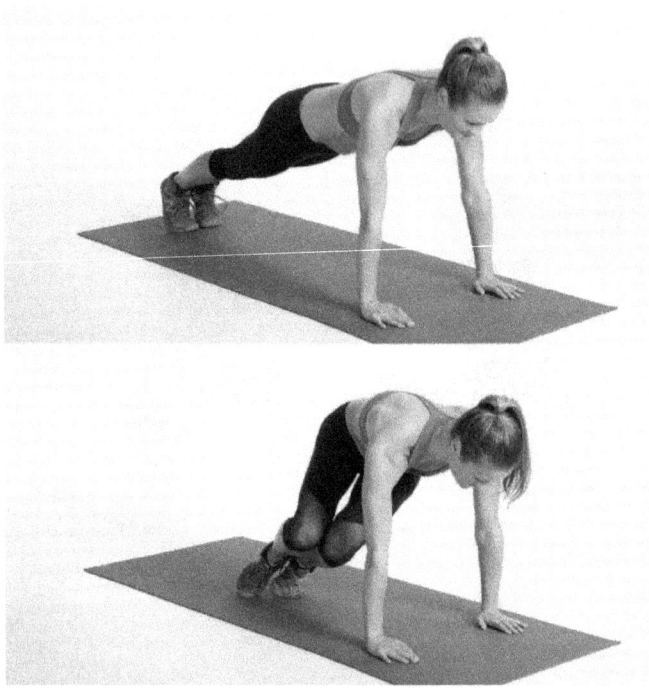

Lay down flat on your stomach. Rise up onto your elbows. Put your palms flat against the floor.

Press your toes into the floor and push up into a plank position. Jump your legs over to your left side while keeping your knees straight and your legs glued together.

Then jump them over to your left side. Repeat.

4. *Falling Towers*

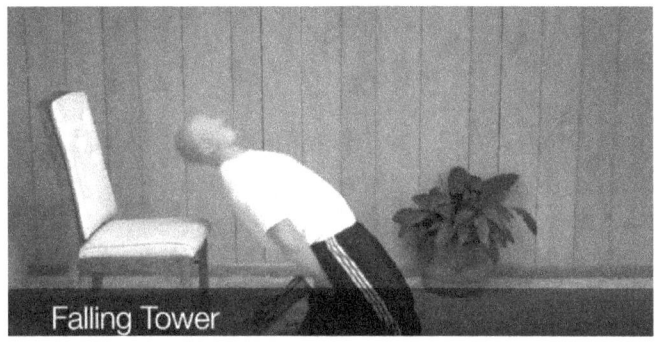

Place a chair behind you. Get into a kneeling position in front of the chair so that your shins and the tops of your feet are flat against the floor.

Lift your thighs up so that your legs form a 90° angle. Clasp your hands behind you so that they hang in front of your butt.

Keep your torso and thighs in one straight line as you lean yourself back until your head just barely touches the seat of the chair. Lift yourself back up. Repeat. You should be using the strength of your thighs to complete this move.

5. *Down Dog with Side Jumps*

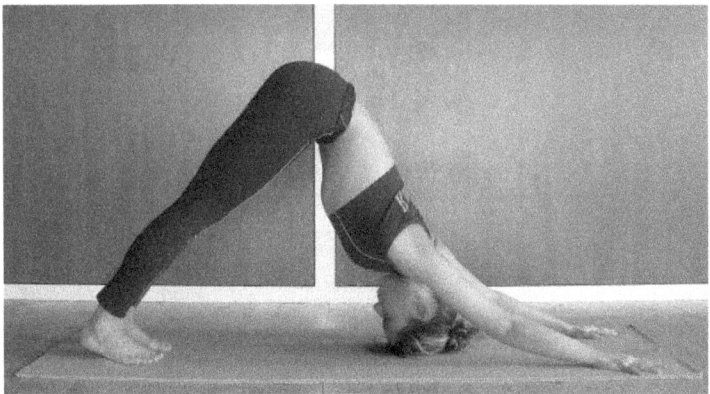

Get into plank position. From this position, lift your butt directly up so that your body forms an upside-down V shape.

Just as with the plank side jumps, jump your feet over to the left and then over to the right. Remember to keep your legs glued together and your knees straight.

Repeat this as many times as you can for the full 60 seconds.

Advanced Leg Carving and Toning Workout #2 (With Equipment)

Equipment Needed: Pull Up Bar, Stool, Chair or Coffee Table

1. ***Hanging Leg Raises***

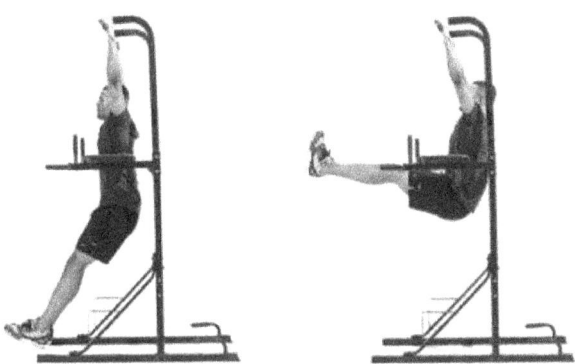

Start by hanging from a pull-up bar. Your arms should be straight but your elbows shouldn't be locked. Keep your legs together and point your toes straight down.

Now lift your legs up while keeping your knees straight and toes pointed. Lift them until they are pointing straight out in front of you.

Lower your legs back down. Repeat this for the full 60 seconds.

2. ***Hanging Bat Sit Ups***

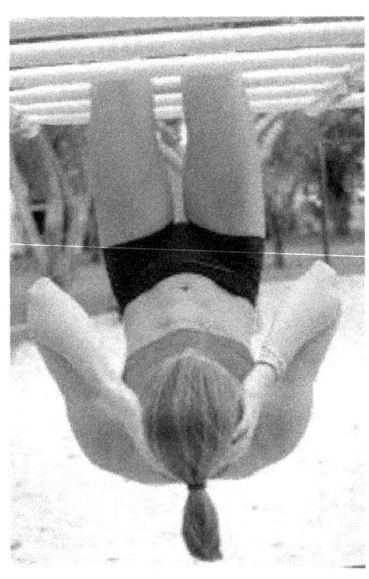

Grab the pull up bar, lift yourself up until your hips are against the pull up bar.

Lift one arm off and put it behind you, twist yourself around and place your free arm back down on the pull up bar so that you are facing away from it.

Sit down on top of the pull up bar. Cross your ankles. Carefully lower yourself down so that you are hanging by your legs. Keep them flexed.

Do sit-ups in this position, pulling your chin all the way to your thighs. Continue this for the full 60 seconds.

3. Hanging Side Kicks

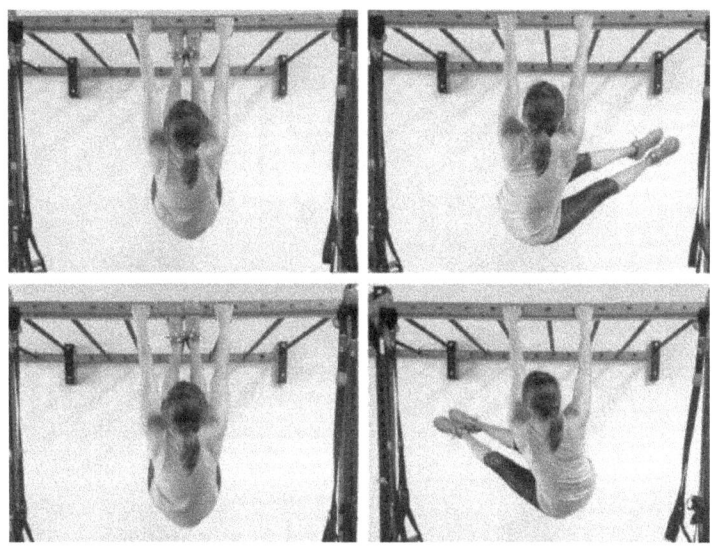

Hang from the pull up bar as you did for the first exercise. Remember not to lock your elbows. Raise your legs out in front of you (again like you did for the first exercise).

Hold them here. Bend both knees to the left side without lowering them down. Kick them out to your left. Bend them back and then return them to the original position straight in front of you.

Repeat this same action on the right side. Continue for 60 seconds.

4. *One Leg Elevated Hip Thrusts*

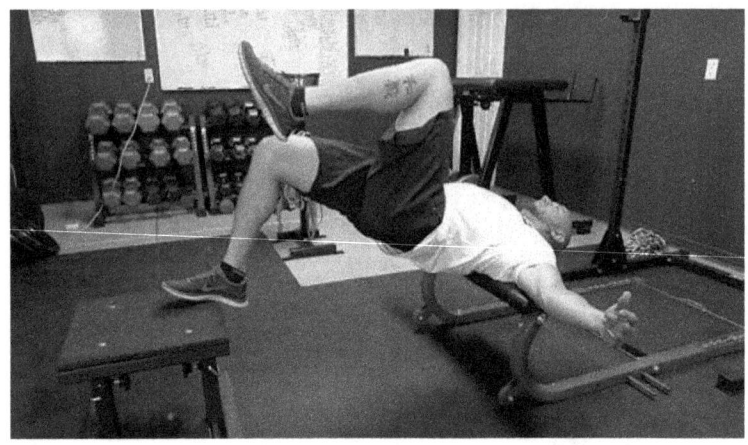

For this, you need a chair or coffee table in front of you and another surface of the same height behind you.

For example, you could do this sitting between your couch and your coffee table.

Place your heels on the edge of the table or chair. Rest your arms on the couch or table behind you. Lift your left leg up in air above the coffee table. Hold it in the air.

With your right leg on the edge of the coffee table, lift your body up until you form a bridge between the table and couch.

Throughout this movement, your left leg should stay raised so that all the effort is coming from your right leg. Lower yourself down. Repeat the exercise with your left leg on the table and your right leg raised. Continue this for 60 seconds.

5. *Plyometric Hops*

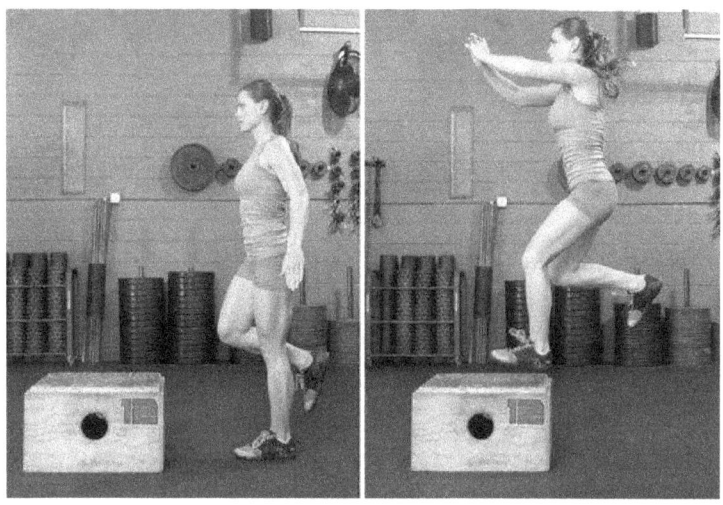

Get a stool that is about 1 to 2 feet high. It should be sturdy and secure so that it doesn't slide around much. You can put it on a carpeted surface to prevent sliding. For this exercise, you will do a series of different jumps. For each jump, your legs should remain together and move in unison.

First, you will jump over it without touching the stool. Turn around, jump back over it.

Turn around, jump onto the stool then jump off on the other side. Turn and then jump onto the stool again. Jump off on the other side. Go to the side of the stool and jump sideways onto the stool.

Jump off to the other side. Then, jump sideways again back onto it. Jump off to the other side.

So, you will repeat: jump over, jump over, jump forward onto it, jump forward onto it, jump sideways onto it, and jump sideways onto it. Repeat this series of jumps for the full 60 seconds.

Advanced Leg Carving and Toning Workout #3 (Cardio Based)

Option 1:

The Treadmill

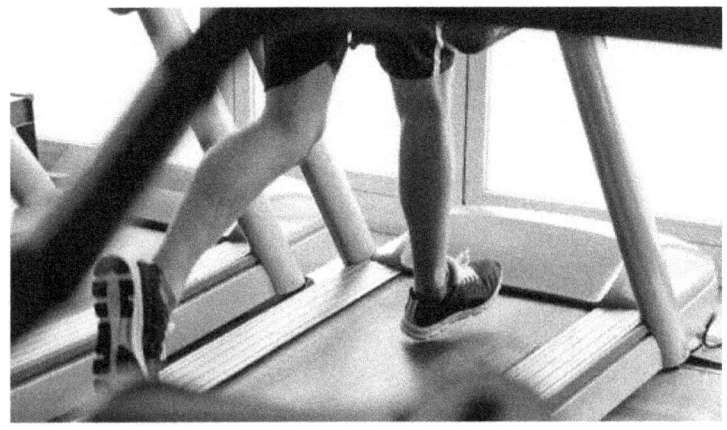

Use a treadmill to do a cardio workout that is fantastic for your legs. Start by running for 40 seconds at your highest possible speed and steepest possible incline.

Then run for 20 seconds at a moderate speed and low incline.

Continue alternating between this high intensity and low intensity running for 15 minutes.

Option 2:

Outdoor Running

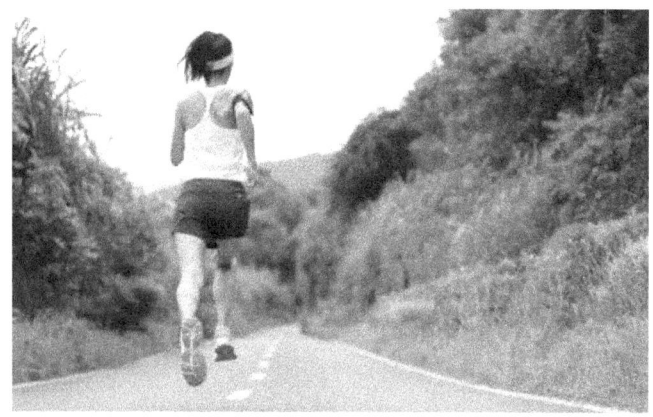

When running outdoors, you won't be able to change the incline at will. One option is to find a hill nearby.

Ideally, it should take you about 40 seconds to run to the top of the hill at your maximum speed. Once at the top, run back down. Repeat this for 15 minutes.

If you live in a flat area and don't have any hills available, just go for a run.

You can alternate between running at your maximum speed for 40 seconds and a moderate speed for 20 seconds. You won't get the full muscle toning benefits of a steep incline but it will still work your muscles.

10 Minute Cool Down

After any of the above workouts, you can use this 10-minute cool down. It is ideal for these workouts because it focuses on stretching your legs (which have just done some intense work and deserve a relaxing stretch):

First, do a little light cardio to help your body transition out of the workout. If you are at a gym, do a low speed walk on the treadmill for 5 minutes.

If you are outdoors, go for a 5-minute walk. If you are at home, just walk around the room for 5 minutes (or take a walk around the block.

After your cool down cardio, you need to do some stretching. Start with a simple forward bend. Keep your legs straight and bend down to touch the floor. Hold this pose for about 30 seconds. Take long, deep breaths while you hold it.

Slowly raise your torso back up until you are standing straight. Walk your legs out to each side so that they form an upside down V shape. Go as wide as you can while maintaining your balance.

Put your hands on your hips and bend forward. Once your torso is parallel with the ground, put your palms on the floor. Sink your head down lower until it touches the floor. If you can't touch the floor, that's okay.

Just go as far down as you can. Hold this for about 30 seconds. Put your hands back on your hips and raise your torso back up. Walk your feet back in until you are standing straight again.

Bend your right foot up and in toward your butt. Grab your ankle with your right hand.

Use your hand to pull your ankle up higher until you can really feel the stretch in the top of your thigh. Let your leg back down and repeat this with your left leg. Do each leg for 30 seconds.

Sit down with your legs out in front of you. Bend your right knee and pull your foot in so that the sole of your foot is pressed against your left inner thigh. Bend forward and wrap your hands around your left foot.

Hold this for 30 seconds while taking slow, deep breaths. Repeat this with your right leg out and your left leg bent.

Lay down on your back with your legs straight. Both feet should be pointed straight out so that your toes are parallel with the floor. Bend the right leg in toward your chest.

Clasp your shin and pull your leg deep into your chest. Remember to keep your toes pointed. Hold this for 30 seconds. Repeat the same move with your left leg.

Sit up in a cross-legged position. Bend forward until your head is touching the ground. Don't let your knees rise up as you bend forward.

Pull them toward the floor. Hold this for 30 seconds. Lift your torso up, cross your legs the other way (so that the bottom leg is now on top).

Bend forward again. Hold for another 30 seconds.

Proven "Fat-Burn" Exercises

Liberty Arabesque

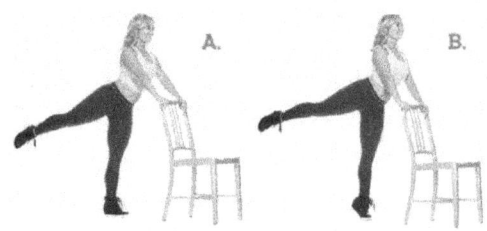

The liberty arabesque can be performed anywhere and at any time. This exercise is highly effective for the lower torso and butt.

Here is how you will do it:

1. Hold onto a chair for balance, standing parallel to the back of the chair.

2. Stand on your tiptoes on one leg and stretch the other out towards the back. Stretch as much as you can. Repeat in sets.

Waist Whittler

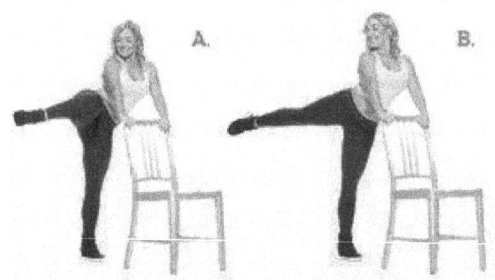

Like the name suggests, this exercise is great for toning your waist.

Here is how you will do it:

1. Maintain your position similar to that of the last exercise, but hold you left feet firmly on the ground.

2. Straining your abs, bend your knee towards the chair and then pull the leg back, stretching it so that it is parallel to the floor. Repeat.

Curtsey to Lateral Liberty

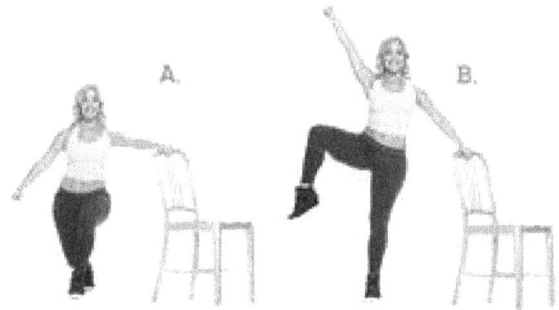

Another extension to the previous two exercises, this one is specially designed to work wonders on your butt.

Here is how you will do it:

1. For this workout, use the positon of your previous workout, pivot to your right holding on to the chair with one hand, inhale and lower into a curtsey lunge.

2. Make a low V with your arms as you reach this posture. Repeat in sets.

The Hip Switch

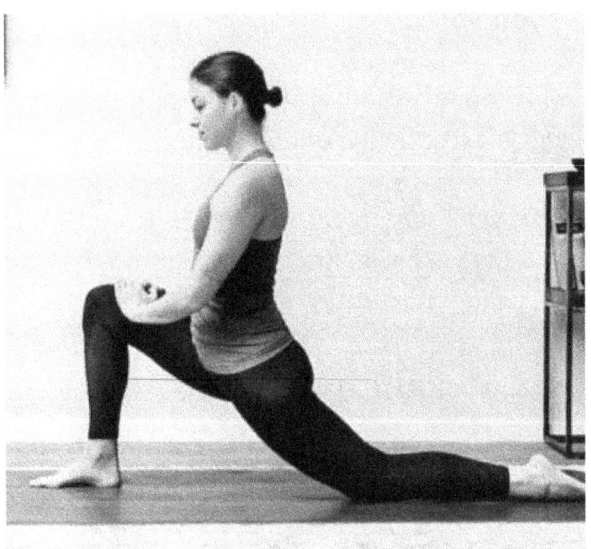

This one is unique and works best for your abs. The hip switch is performed with dumbbells.

Here is how you will do it:

1. Stand tall. Then lower your right leg slightly below hip height and reach it long towards the floor. Inhale and use your abs to rotate your hips.

2. Then turn your glutes towards the sky while exhaling. Repeat this exercise with the other leg.

Gurney

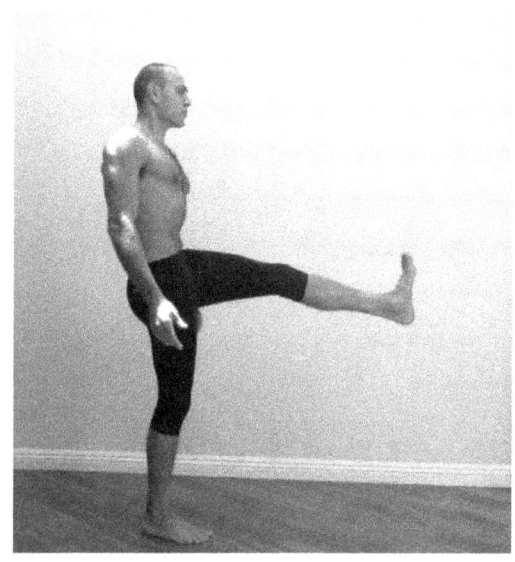

The gurney will help build your entire core, especially the thighs and hips.

Here is how you will do it:

1. Stand tall and then keeping your legs straight; try to reach the floor with your arms.

2. Lift your right leg straight up, stretching as far as you can. Repeat the same with the other leg.

Pick Up

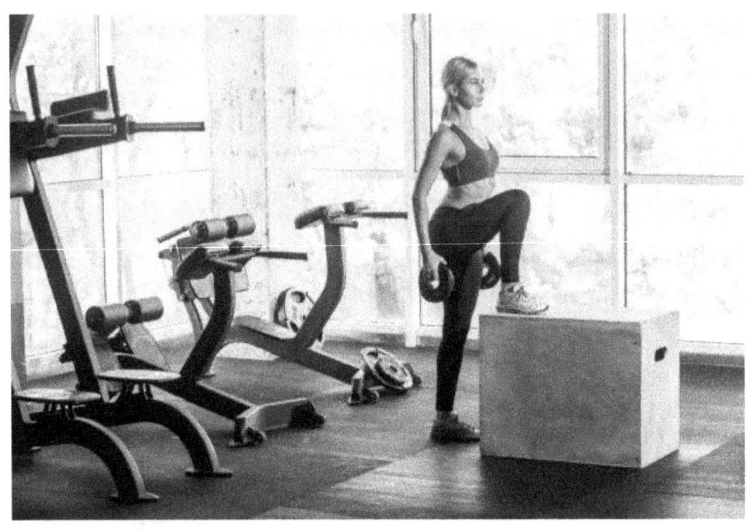

This unique exercise is designed so you can get the most out of the exercise in as little time as possible. The pick-up is performed with the help of a chair for best results.

Here is how you will do it:

1. Start by standing in front of the chair, such that you are facing away from it.

2. Now, balance on your right leg as you place your left toe on the chair. Make sure you keep your legs straight.

3. Pick up your dumbbells and stretch your arms towards the ceiling. Relax and repeat with the other leg.

Turning the Pyramid

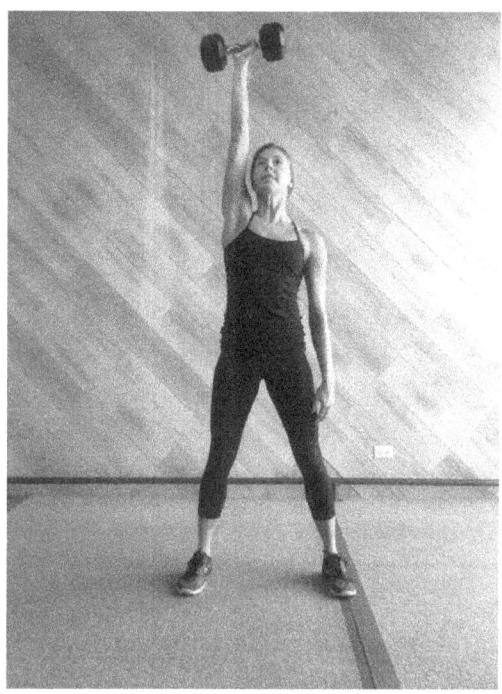

Turning the pyramid is performed while standing up. You can increase the intensity of this workout by holding a pair of dumbbells in your hands.

Here is how you will do it:

1. Take your position by standing tall. Balance on left leg with right leg lifted behind you and arms out to sides;

2. Exhale and pivot to the right as you lift your right leg toward the ceiling and out to the side. Repeat in sets.

Star

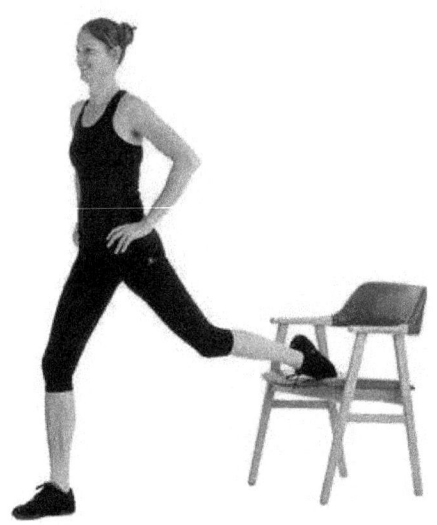

The star is performed using the chair for support. This one is ideal for the waist and hips.

Here is how you will do it:

1. Pivot to your right with you left leg stretched out on a chair. Keep the other leg straight.

2. Stretch your arms wide apart until they are at shoulder length, parallel to the ground. Keeping your lower body pivoted in the same position, try to reach the ground with your right fingertips.

3. Relax back to the original position and then repeat. Hold some weight in your hand to give yourself a little challenge.

Pike up

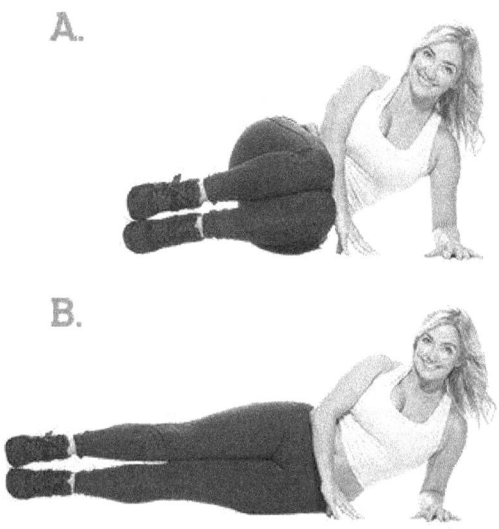

A.

B.

The pike up is an excellent variation to the hips and waist exercises. Performed without any dumbbells or stability balls, this one can be performed anywhere at any time.

To challenge yourself, adjust the weight of the dumbbells in your hand. Ideally, start with five pounds and then work your way towards ten pounds.

Here is how you will do it:

1. Lie on the floor sideways, on your hips, resting your upper body on your elbows, palm planted to the floor. Inhale and tuck your knees towards your chest.

2. Now, exhale and stretch your legs out such that your body is in one line. Pike up now, with your legs and one arm forming a deep V. Repeat.

Split to Toe Touch

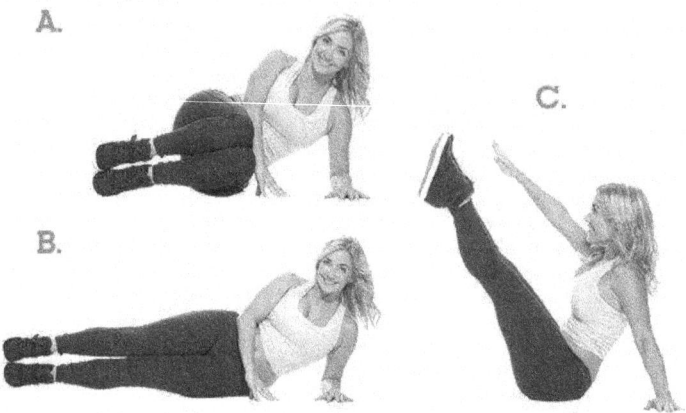

Another simple variation to the pike up, this one will work on your lower abs and thighs.

Here is how you will do it:

1. Start with your initial position in pike up and swing your legs forwards alternately to the sides, without touching the floor.

2. Pivot 90 degrees and stretch your legs to the ceiling. Now split your legs. Repeat.

Pike Kick

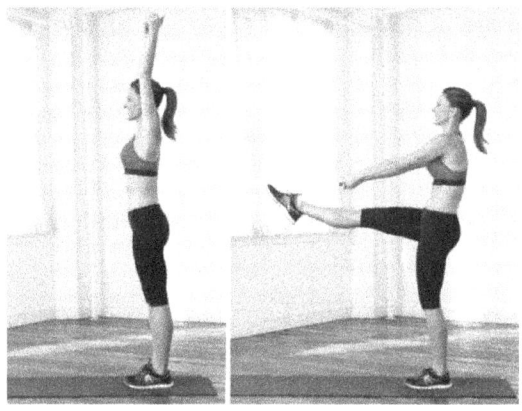

The pick tick tones your torso and your thighs, tightening the butt.

Here is how you will do it:

1. Holding a weight in your hands, stand straight with your arms stretched out on top of you.

2. Now, as you stretch your legs out so that they are parallel to the floor, bring both your hand to touch your thighs. Make sure you don't bend your arms or your legs. Repeat.

Reverse Lunge with Twist and Pull

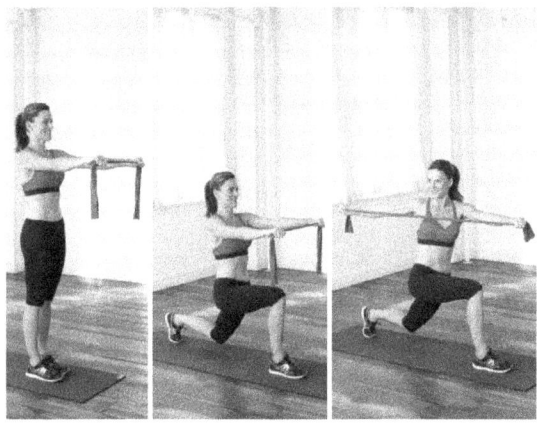

This reverse lunge will work on your core and your back, especially your abs.

Here is how you will do it:

1. Stand straight with your arms extended in front of you so that they are parallel to the floor.

2. Use a band in your hands and as you stretch your left leg backwards, twist your torso over to the right as you stretch out your left arms clockwise. Repeat.

Cardio Burst

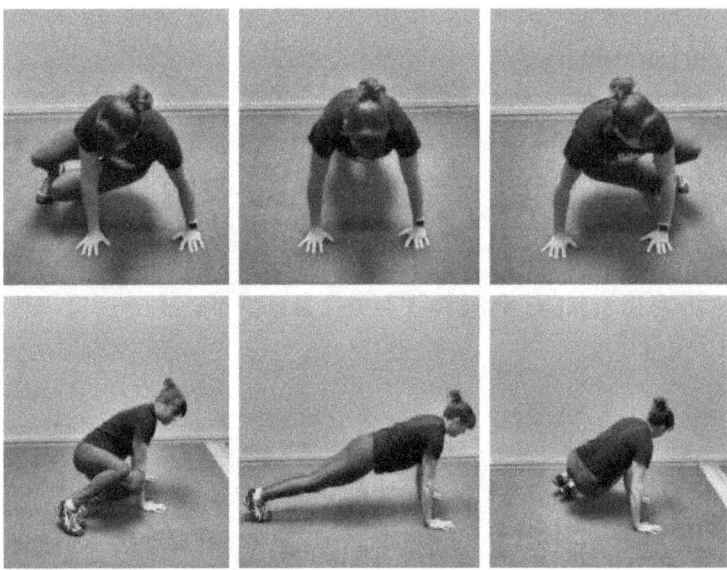

The cardio burst works on the entire core, your chest and your shoulders and you will lose weight in no time.

Here is how you will do it:

1. Get down to the regular push up position, with your arms straight and your feet together.

2. Now hop your foot out on either side. Repeat.

Squat Punch

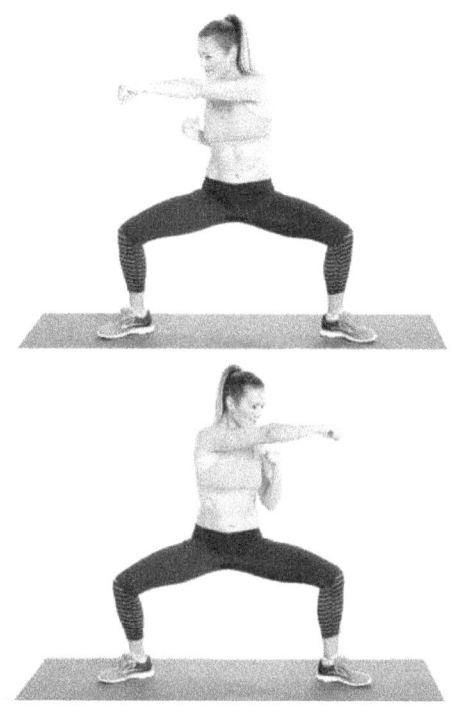

The squat punch is very effective for the butt and the waist. To challenge yourself, adjust the weight of the dumbbells in your hand. Ideally, start with five pounds and then work your way towards ten pounds.

Here is how you will do it:

1. Stand with feet slightly more than hip-width apart, 1 weight in each hand. Raise the weights to shoulders length, with your palms facing forward.

2. Lower into a squat position. Extend left arms at shoulder length. Repeat with the other hand.

Side-Angle Bent Row

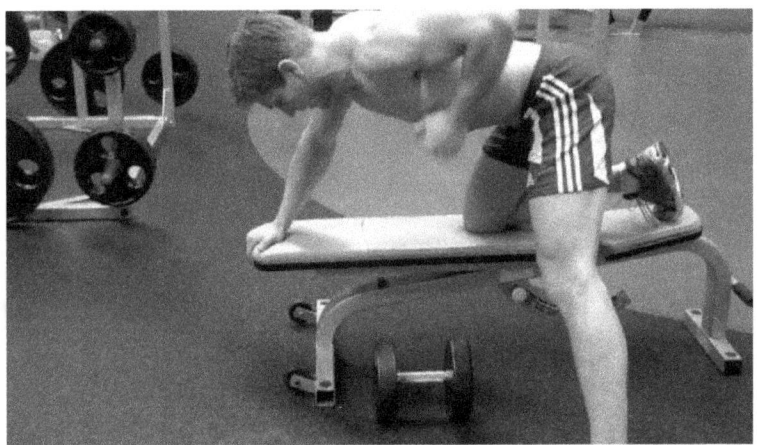

The side-angle bent row is ideal for the butt and the lower back.

Here is how you will do it:

1. Using a band, anchor it under the inside of your feet.

2. Bend your left foot back so that it is parallel to the ground. Lower your right hand next to the left shin, next move your right elbow towards your left shoulder. Repeat.

3. For variation, use dumbbells instead of the band and vary the weight to challenge yourself.

Plank Walk-in

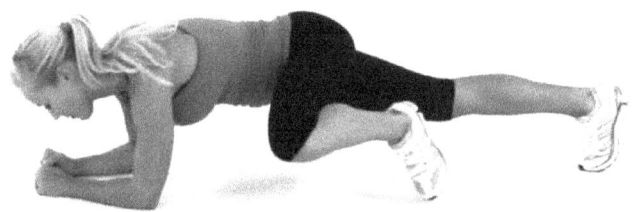

This simple exercise is specifically designed for the butt, the thighs and the waist.

Here is how you will do it:

1. Start by assuming the push up position, keeping your arms straight. Stressing your core, push your left foot towards your left arm and vice versa coming to a squat position. Repeat.

2. For variation, add some weigh to the exercise, use dumbbells and then adjust the weight of the dumbbells in your hand. Ideally, start with five pounds and then work your way towards ten pounds.

Plank Hip Dip

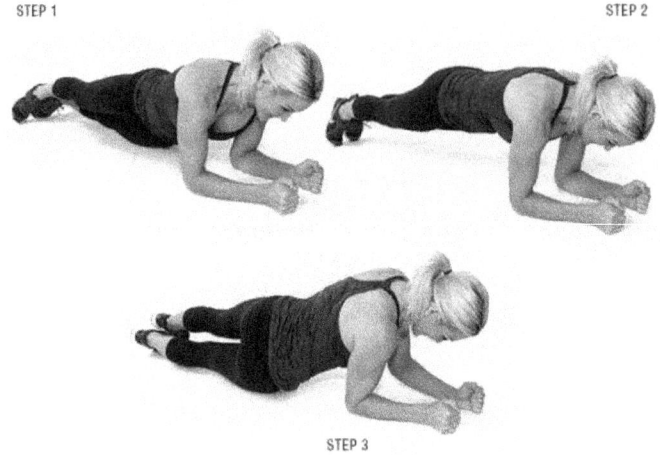

The plank hip dip will work on everything, from the shoulders to your entire core, giving you the body you have been dying for.

Here is how you will do it:

1. Stand with the forearm plank with your elbows under your shoulders.

2. Stressing for core for the impact, twist your hips so that you right hip touches the floor slightly. Repeat on the opposite side.

3. Complete in sets of two, each set of twenty reps at least.

Boat with T-Row

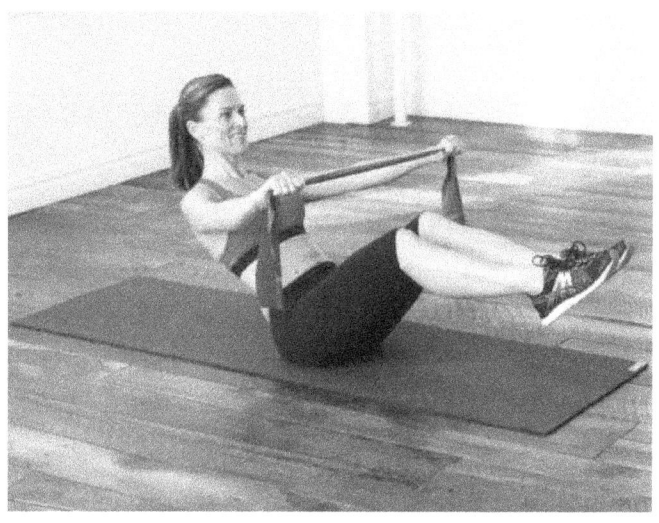

This exercise is specially designed to help you with you back and your shoulder muscles. It also works on the hips and the thighs.

Here is how you will do it:

1. Assume your position by placing your feet right on the floor and knees bent as you assume the seated position.

2. Use a band that you will hold on each hand.

3. Lift your feet of the floor and try to balance on your hip bones, pulling your hand apart to stretch the band as far as you can. Repeat in sets.

The Glute Kick

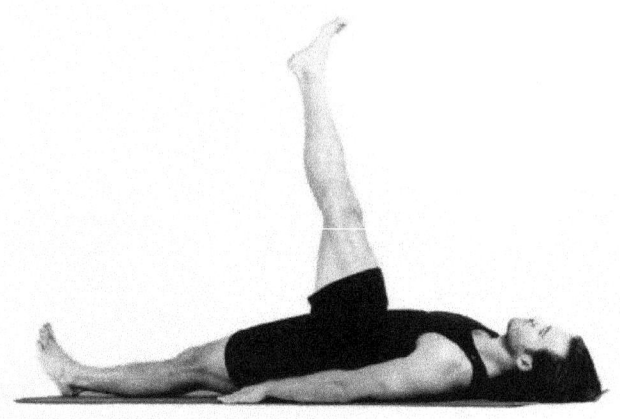

The glute kick is specially designed for the butt and the thighs and especially your core.

This one is simple and gives quick results.

Here is how you will do it:

1. For this exercise, you will need to lie back and with your left knee bend, extend your right knee straight above the ground.

2. Continue lifting your leg and then releasing it for around thirty seconds; repeat the same with the other exercises.

Bird Dog Crunch

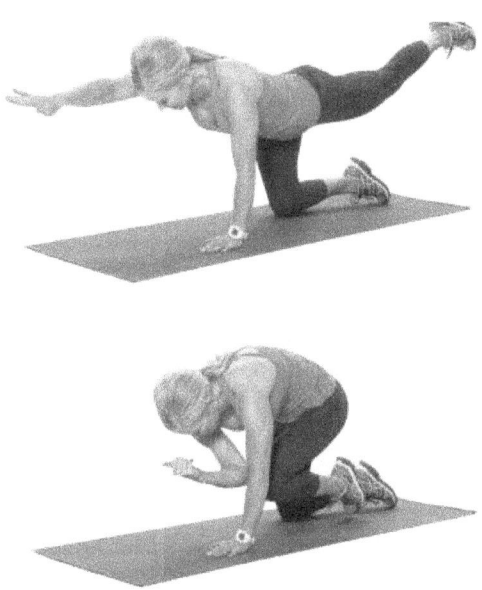

Performed on all fours, this is another effective exercise that will give immediate results.

Here is how you will do it:

1. Start by standing on all fours. Hold a five-pound weight in the left hand.

2. Stressing your core, bend your right leg backwards and right arm forward with your hand on the floor, palm down. You should now be in a starting position. Repeat the exercise with the other leg. Perform the exercise in sets.

3. To challenge yourself, adjust the weight of the dumbbells in your hand. Ideally, start with five pounds and then work your way towards ten pounds.

The Superman Pull

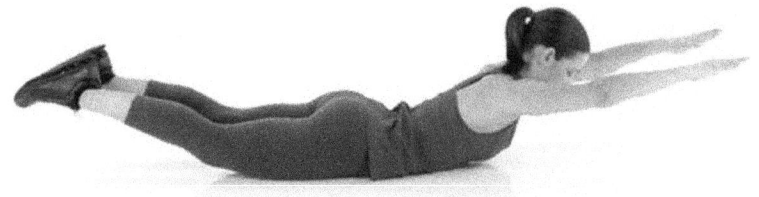

The superman pull is especially designed for busy women who want to get the best out of a few minutes of exercise.

Here is how you will do it:

1. Lie on the floor, face down, with your arms extending above your head. Slowly lift your arms, your legs and your chest a few inches above your body, bringing your elbows towards your chest.

2. Return to starting positon and begin again. Repeat in sets of two.

Single Leg Hip Raise

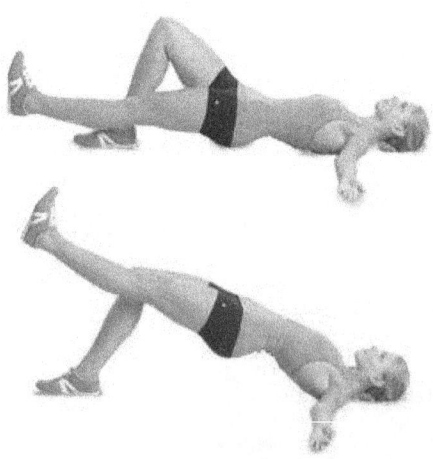

Performed while lying on the floor, this hip exercise will give you results in a matter of minutes.

Here is how you will do it:

1. Lie on you back, facing the ceiling with your legs slightly bent, hands stretched out on either side, away from the body.

2. Lift your hips above the ground with your feet on the ground. Stretch as much as you can

3. Alternately, raise your legs as high as you can, one at a time. Repeat in sets.

Marching Hip Raise

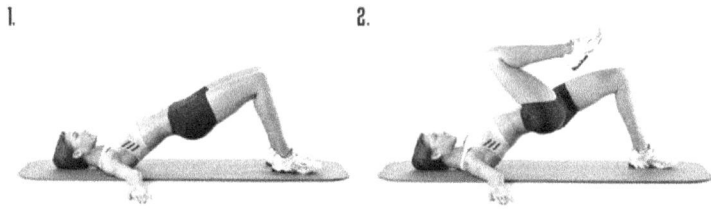

Another one, similar to the single leg hip raise, this one is also designed to work on your butt and your abs simultaneously.

Here is how you will do it:

1. Lie on you back, facing the ceiling with your legs slightly bent, hands stretched out on either side, away from the body.

2. Lift your hips above the ground with your feet on the ground.

3. Now, pull your right leg towards your chest. Do the same with the other leg. Repeat in sets of twenty each.

Swiss Ball Hips Raise and Leg Curl

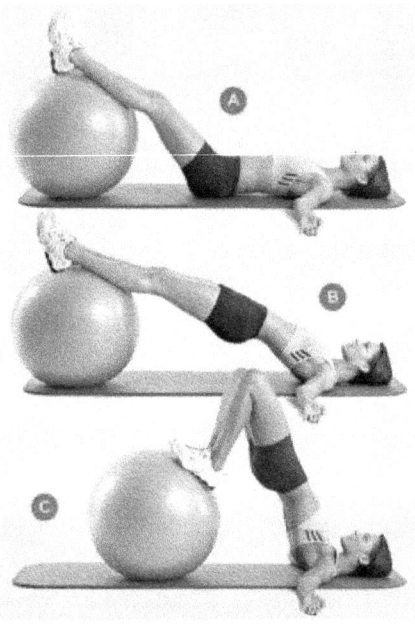

This exercise is performed with the help of a stability ball. The Swiss ball hips raise and curl works on your hips, your thighs and your torso.

Here is how you will do it:

1. Lie on you back, facing the ceiling with your legs slightly bent, hands stretched out on either side, away from the body.

2. Lift your hips above the ground with your feet resting on the stability ball.

3. Now, roll the ball as close to your butt while pulling the stability ball towards you with the hells of your feet.

Barbell Deadlift

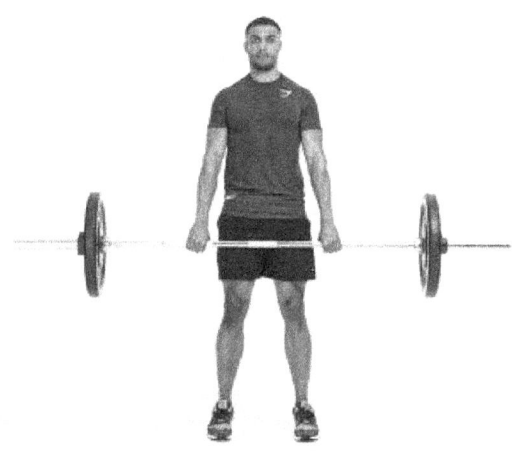

Performed using a barbell, this one is designed to tone your butt and your thighs.

Here is how you will do it:

1. Stand tall and hold onto the loaded barbells in an overhand grip. Make sure your hands are just below your shoulders. Put the barbell back down and raise it again. Repeat.

2. To challenge yourself, adjust the weight of the barbells in your hand. Ideally, start with five pounds and then work your way towards ten pounds.

Dumbbell Deadlift

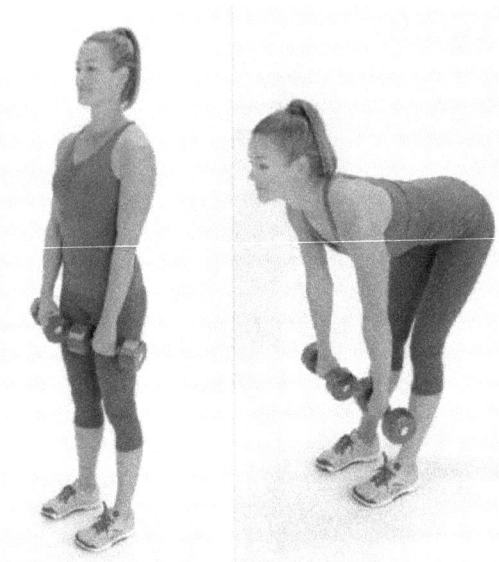

This exercise is a variation of the barbell deadlift, performed while using the dumbbell instead of the barbell.

Here is how you will do it:

1. Stand tall and hold onto the dumbbells, one in each hand, in an overhand grip. Make sure your hands are just below your shoulders.

2. Put the dumbbells back down and raise them again. Repeat.

3. To increase the intensity of the exercise, play with different weights of the barbells. Start with three pounds and then work your way towards ten.

Single Leg Deadlift

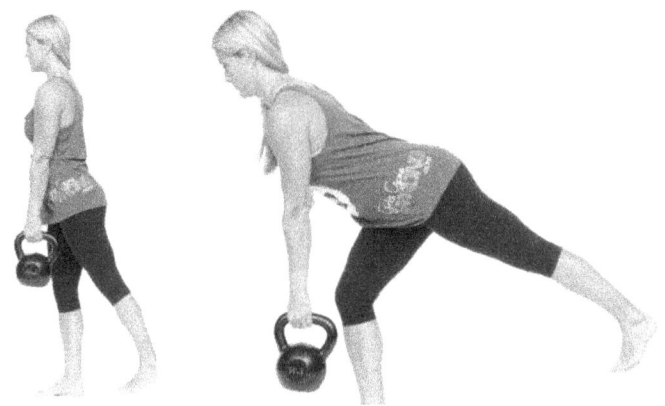

Single leg deadlift is another variation of the previous two exercises, except that it is performed without any weight.

Here is how you will do it:

1. Stand tall with your arms on the side. Keep your palms open. Make sure your hands are just below your shoulders

2. Now, balance on one leg for around 30 second while bending down with one leg. Repeat the same with the other leg.

3. To challenge yourself, add weight to your hands using dumbbells. Adjust the weight of the dumbbells in your hand. Ideally, start with five pounds and then work your way towards ten pounds.

Single Arm Dumbbell Swing

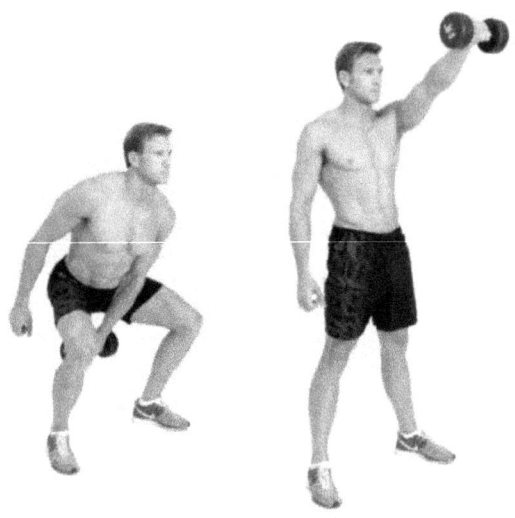

This one uses dumbbell for toning your butt and shoulders.

Here is how you will do it:

1. Stand tall and hold onto the dumbbells, one in each hand, in an overhand grip. Make sure your hands are just below your shoulders. Push your legs wide apart.

2. Swing the dumbbells in between your legs and then straight ahead, stretch your arms straight while you complete your pose. Repeat the exercise with the other hand.

3. To challenge yourself, adjust the weight of the dumbbells in your hand. Ideally, start with five pounds and then work your way towards ten pounds.

Clamshell

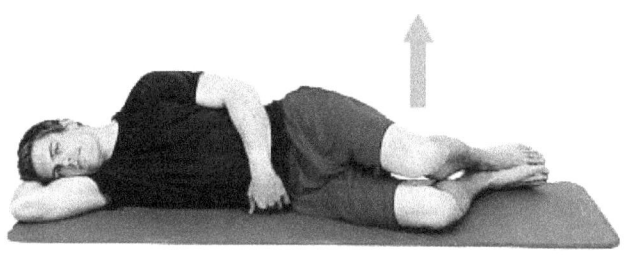

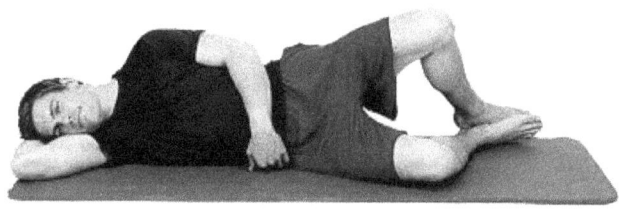

The clamshell is performed while lying to your side. Works best on your thighs and butt.

Here is how you will do it:

1. Lie on your side with you left arms beneath your head.

2. Staying in one position you should lift your right leg above the ground keeping your pelvis constant. Hold yourself in that position for a few seconds. Relax and repeat.

Dumbbell Step-up

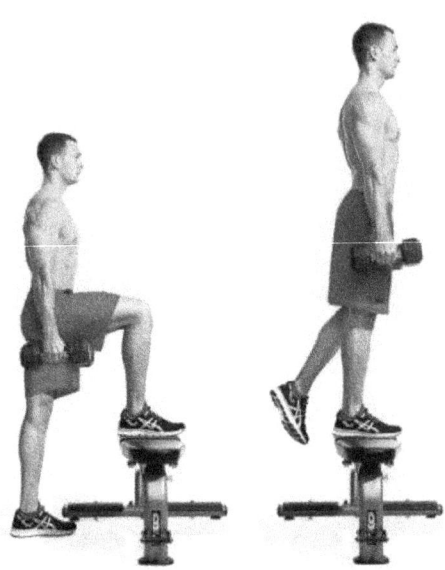

Using a step, this exercise is designed to work on your abs and your shoulder, also works on your thighs and butt.

Here is how you will do it:

1. Stand tall and hold onto the dumbbells, one in each hand, in an overhand grip. Make sure your hands are just below your shoulders.

2. Now, step on the step one at a time. Repeat.

3. To challenge yourself, adjust the weight of the dumbbells in your hand. Ideally, start with five pounds and then work your way towards ten pounds.

The Plank

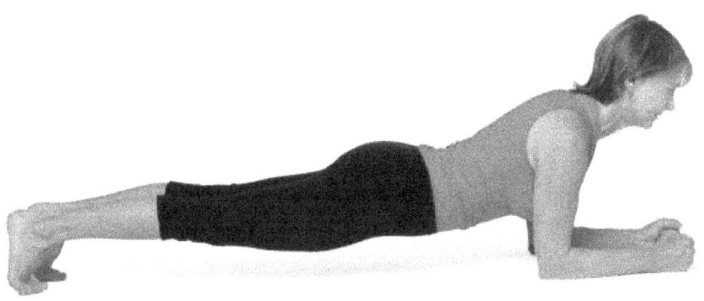

Especially designed to work on your lower and your upper abs, this one is performed without any balls or barbells.

Here is how you will do it:

1. Start with the push up position and rest your upper body on your elbows.

2. Make sure your body forms a straight line from your shoulders to your ankles. Hold and then repeat.

Plank to Push Up

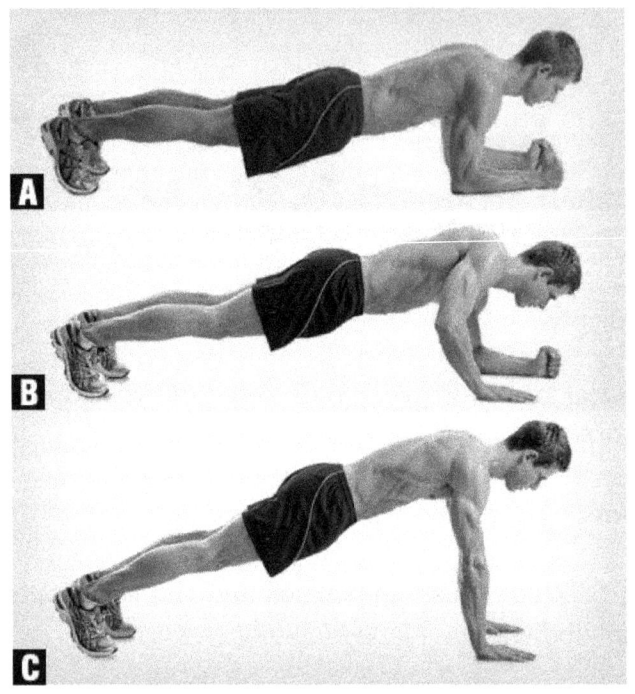

A variation to the plank, this one is easy and effective.

Here is how you will do it:

1. Start with the push up position and rest your upper body on your elbows. Make sure your body forms a straight line from your shoulders to your ankles.

2. Push up, stretching your arms straight. Repeat.

Plank Jumping Jacks

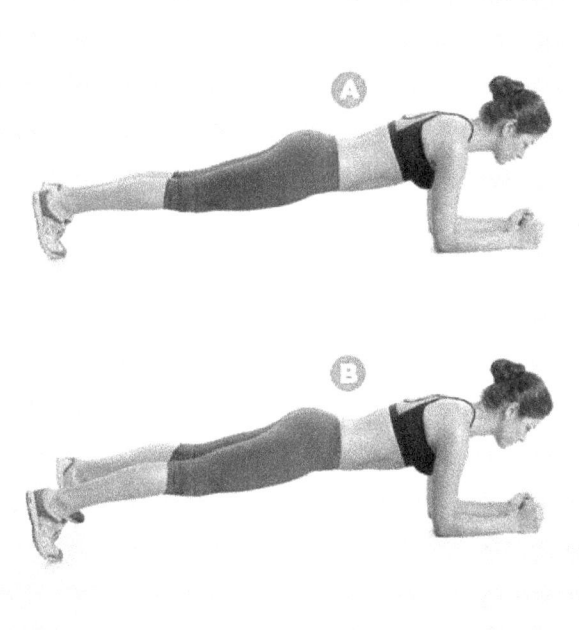

This one is specially designed to work on your butts and your thighs.

Here is how you will do it:

1. Start with the push up position and rest your upper body on your elbows. Make sure your body forms a straight line from your shoulders to your ankles.

2. Jump your legs apart and then jump them back again. Repeat.

Plank with Arm Extension

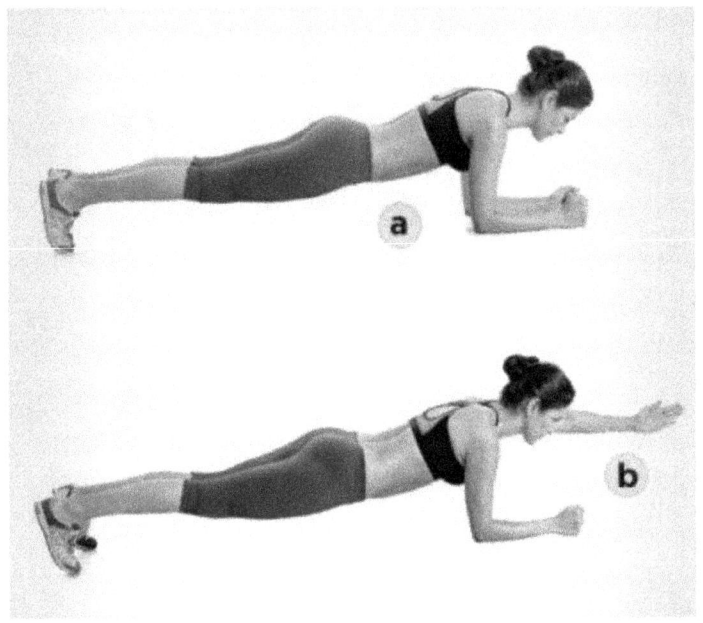

Performed using the same plank position, this one stresses the toning of your arms and your waistline.

Here is how you will do it:

1. Start with the push up position and rest your upper body on your elbows. Make sure your body forms a straight line from your shoulders to your ankles.

2. Stretch one arm forward until it is parallel to the ground. Repeat.

Rolling Plank

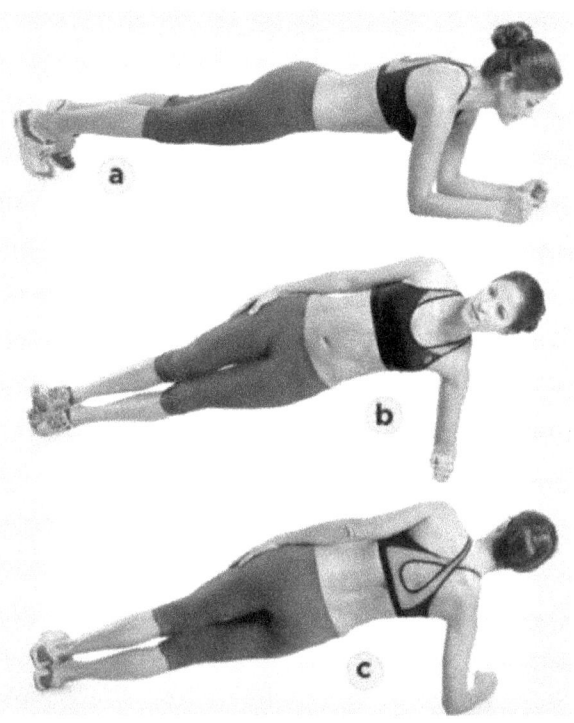

Another exercise that is best for your thighs, your butt and your abs. This one can be performed anywhere, at any time, without any prop.

Here is how you will do it:

1. Begin with the basic plank position, and then shift into a side plank.

2. Do the same on the other side. Stretch your arms upwards. Repeat and complete in sets.

Side Plank and Rotate

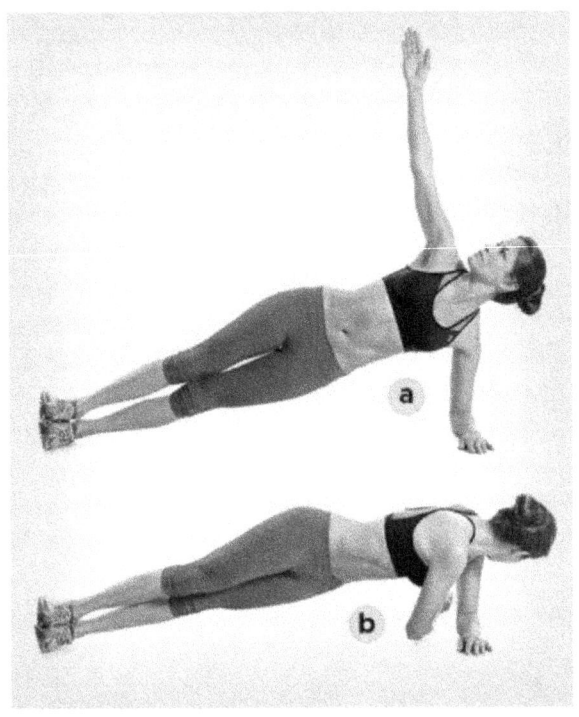

This exercise is performed using the side plank position. This is an excellent variation to the traditional plank pose.

Here is how you will do it:

1. Start with the push up position and rest your upper body on your elbows. Make sure your body forms a straight line from your shoulders to your ankles. Then twist to the side plank position.

2. Try to reach in between the space of your body with the hand on the opposite side. Repeat.

Planking Frog Tucks

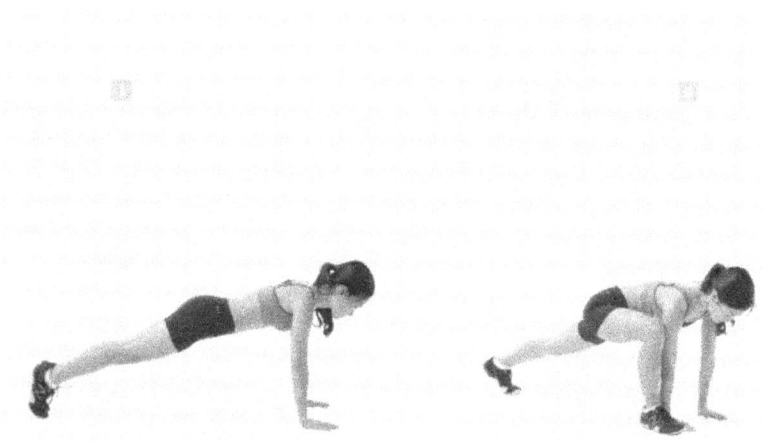

The planking frog tucks is another variation to the basic plank position that helps lose the extra flabs on your butt in no time.

Here is how you will do it:

1. Start with the push up position and rest your upper body on your elbows. Make sure your body forms a straight line from your shoulders to your ankles.

2. Bring one knee towards your torso one at a time, stretching as much as you can. Try to keep the other leg as straight as possible. Repeat.

Swiss Ball Plank with Feet on Bench

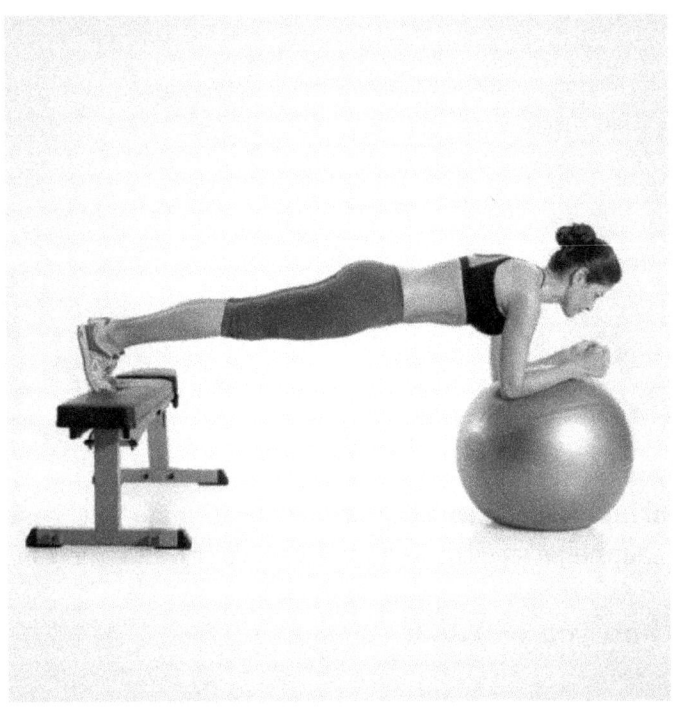

Performed using the step and the Swiss ball, this unique exercise helps tone your body fast and quick.

Here is how you will do it:

1. Start with the push up position and rest your upper body on the Swiss ball. Stabilize on the ball with your elbows.

2. Place your feet on the step. Hold onto this position for a while and then repeat.

Body Weight Jump Squat

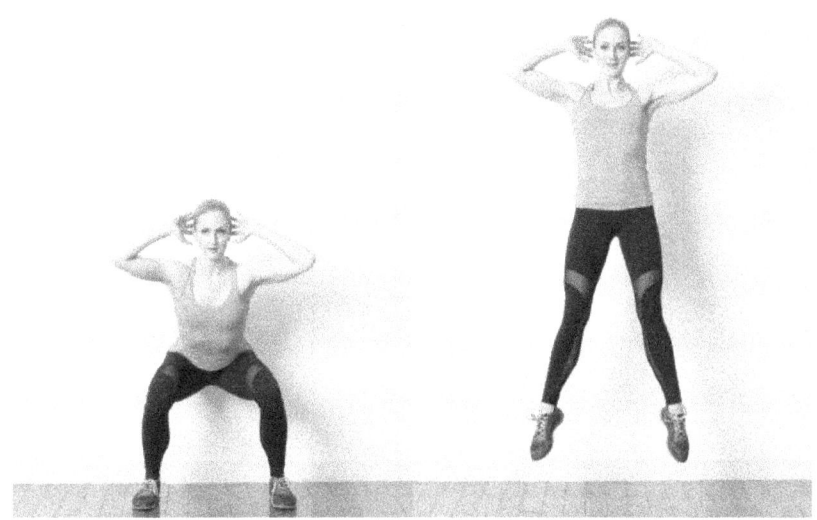

Performed without any weights, this is an easy exercise that works your butt and your thighs.

Here is how you will do it:

1. Stand firmly, legs shoulder-width apart, hands behind your head. Make sure your elbows are aligned to each other and they are parallel to the ground.

2. Maintaining that position, jump as high as you can, keeping your legs straight. After you return to your position, repeat the same step again. Repeat.

3. To challenge yourself, use dumbbells and adjust the weight of the dumbbells in your hand. Ideally, start with five pounds and then work your way towards ten pounds.

Pistol Squat

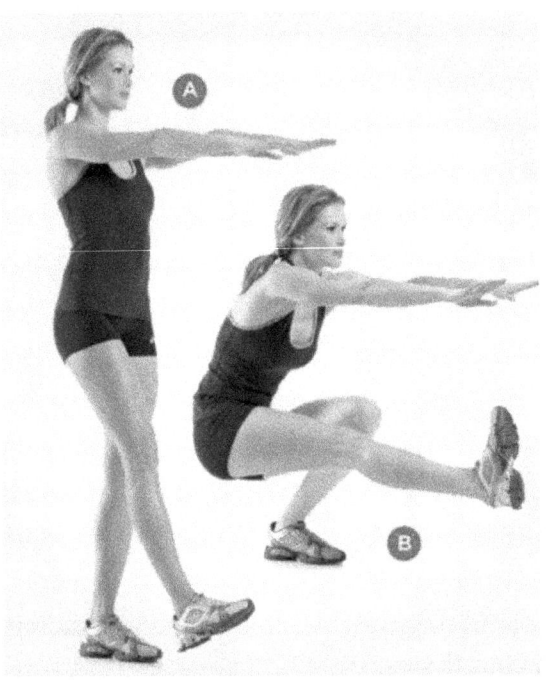

Another exercise that does not use any weights, this can be performed anywhere at any time. The pistol squat is a very easy way to work your butt and your thighs.

Here is how you will do it:

1. Stand firmly, legs shoulder-width apart, hands behind your head.

2. Stretch your legs in the front. Try to make them parallel the ground. Then use the other leg. Repeat.

3. To challenge yourself, hold a pair of dumbbells to the exercise and adjust the weight of the dumbbells in your hand. Ideally, start with five pounds and then work your way towards ten pounds.

Wide Stance Barbell Squat

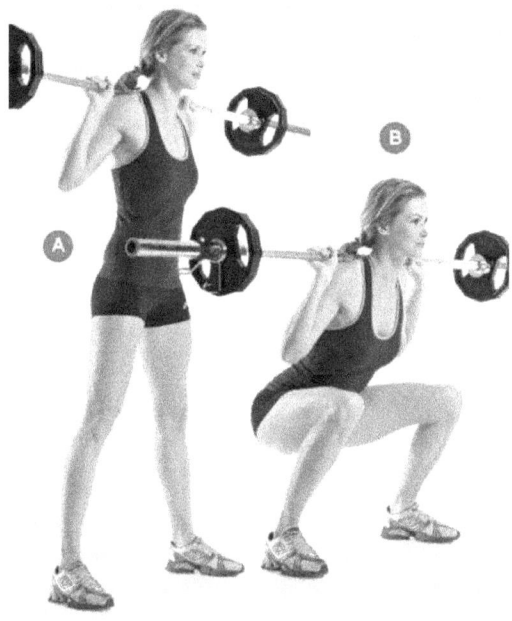

The wide stance barbell squat is another butt exercise that uses barbell to add intensity to the exercise and help you lose your weight fast.

Here is how you will do it:

1. Stand firmly on the ground, with your feet planted firmly to the ground. Make sure your feet are more than your shoulder-width apart.

2. Pull up the barbell and place the barbell behind your head, palms facing the ceiling. Now squat. Repeat the exercise.

3. If you want to increase the intensity of the exercise, add different weights to the barbells and challenge yourself.

Split Squat and Stability Ball

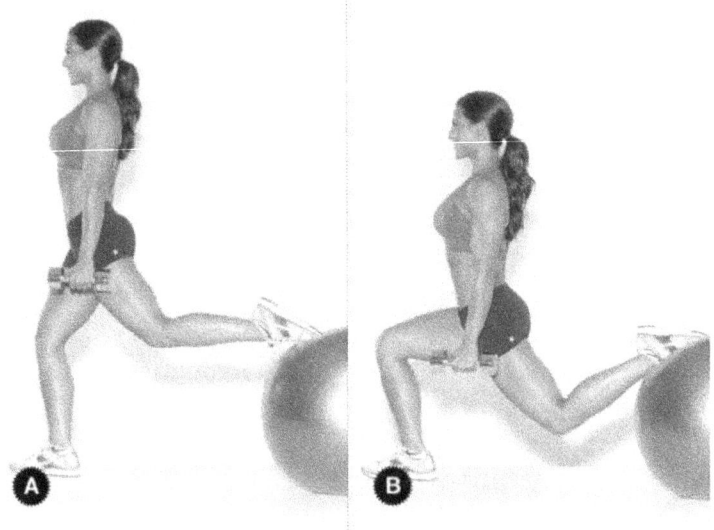

This simple exercise works on your belly like no other exercise. This exercise uses a stability ball for the chore. An excellent exercise that will work on your quadriceps and hamstrings while helping you get a flat stomach.

Here is how you will do it:

1. Stand at a stride's distance from the stability ball. Place the top of the right foot and your shin on the ball.

2. Next, you need to bend your left legs at an angle of 90 degrees while keeping the keeping the knee aligned with your ankle. Then try to straighten the left leg.

3. If you want to challenge yourself a little bit, use a few pounds of dumbbells in your hands and then do the exercise. To modify the exercise a little bit, place the stability ball against a wall and repeat exercise.

One and One-Fourth Push-up

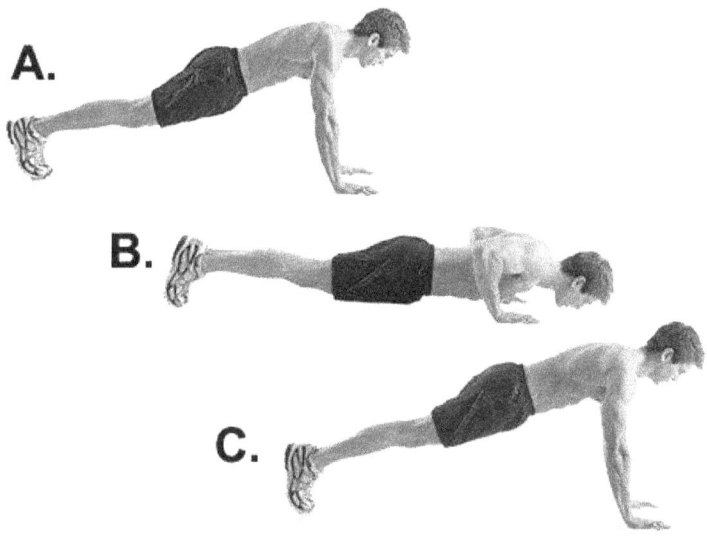

This is another easy, yet challenging exercise. You don't need any stability ball or dumbbells for this one. Start doing this exercise anywhere at any time. This one is an effective exercise that will give you immediate results.

Here is how you will do it:

1. Get down to your regular push up position. Bend your elbows at an angle of 90 degrees and lower your body towards the floor, counting till three every time.

2. Now get back up one quarter of the way and then go down again without touching the floor.

3. Complete the set by going all the way up and then start again.

Torso Twist on Stability Ball

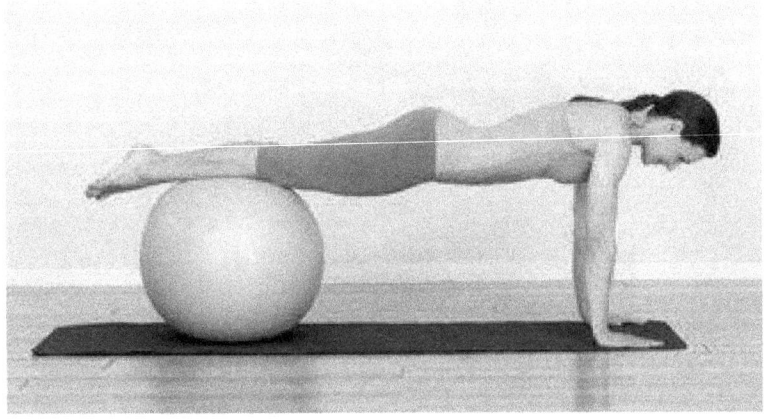

An ideal exercise for development of abs. This one will give you instant result. It uses the basic twist and combines it with the stability ball to invent an amazing ab exercise.

Here is how you will do it:

1. You will start with the regular push up position for this exercise. Make sure your palms are aligned with your shoulders for an upright position.

2. Next, you will lower your feet to the sides of the stability ball. Using this position, keeping your upper body in place, move you lower body to your left and then your right.

3. If you want you can keep your knees to either sides of the ball and then twist.

Back Extension on Stability Ball

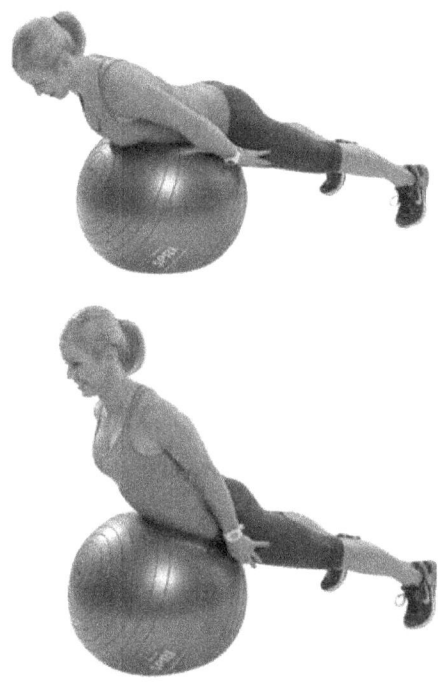

A very good exercise for your lower back, this exercise works wonders to your exercise regimen. This exercise is especially useful if you want a fat belly. Performed with a simple stability ball, this one can be easily performed in a little space.

Here is how you will do it:

1. Start by lying face down on your stability ball, rest your hips on the ball and keep your feet on the floor.

2. Lift your upper body from the ball, keeping your lower body in the same position. Continue by coming back to the starting position.

3. For variation, rest your feet on the wall and redo the entire exercise.

Standing Dumbbell Curl

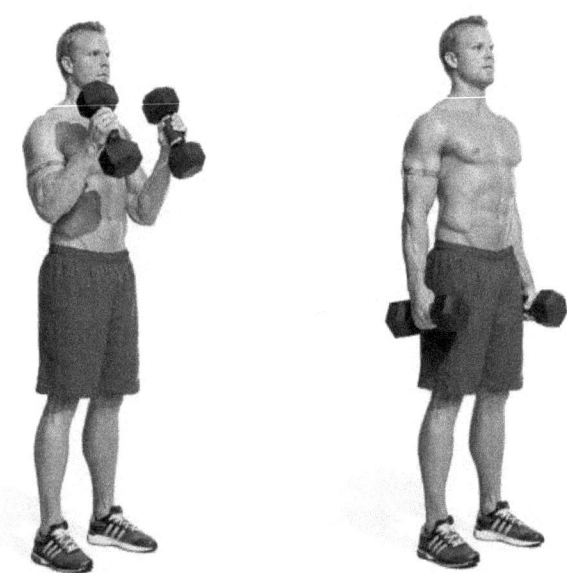

This exercise will work wonders on your shoulders and biceps and help you achieve your perfect body with a flattened to-die-for belly. No stability ball for this one. All you need is a pair of dumbbells and you are good to go.

Here is how you will do it:

1. Stand tall with your feet shoulder-width apart. Now, you will perform your exercise using this position, using a five-pound dumbbell. If you find it comfortable, go as high as ten pounds with your dumbbells.

2. Keeping your arms straight on your sides, curl your dumbbells on your way to the shoulders.

3. For variation, you can also fan your elbows out to the sides, making sure the palms are facing forward. Then turn your elbows at an angle of ninety degrees and perform the exercise.

Medicine Dumbbell Pullover

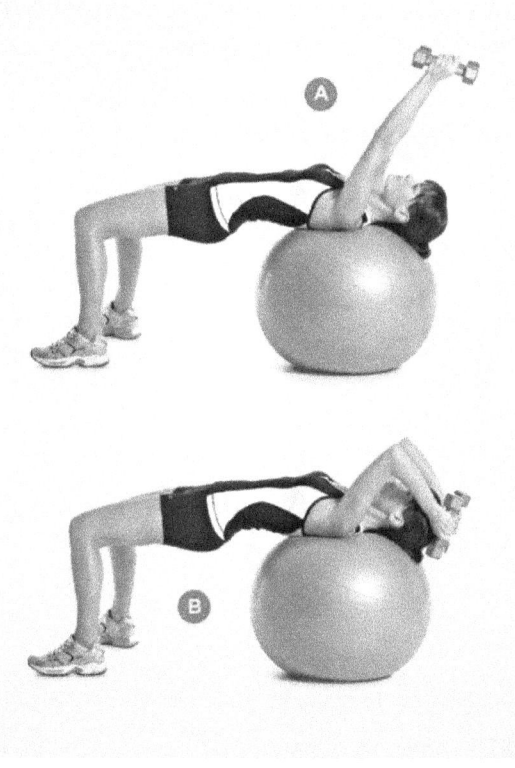

This exercise is perfect for your abs. Performed with a pair of dumbbells, this one is ideal if you are looking to make some abs. This one is a classic twist to the traditional medicine dumbbell pullover and it is more specifically called the one and one-fourth medicine ball pullover.

Here is how you will do it:

1. For this exercise, you will need to lie on a flat surface, such that your feet touch the floor.

2. Now, hold the dumbbells in your hands and stretch your hands straight above your shoulders.

3. Return your hands towards your chest, shopping one fourth of the way down, then go back up. Continue this exercise in sets of ten and move to twenty-five.

Traditional Military Press

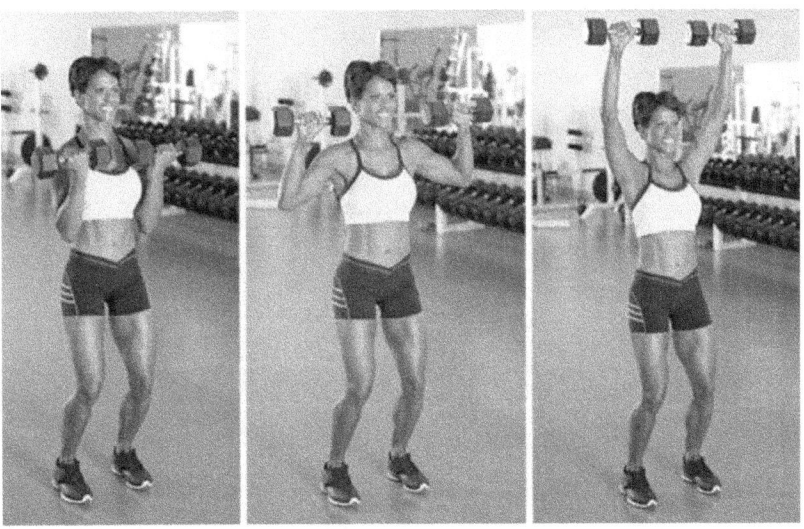

A very traditional, yet, very effective exercise is vital in your exercise regimen. It will add variety to your exercise routine and provide effective results in less than two weeks.

Here is how you will do it:

1. Start this exercise by first taking your position. Stand straight up holding the dumbbells in your hands.

2. Now, stretch your hands directly above your shoulders until your arms are straight. Next, you will rotate your palms so they face inwards. Return your palms to the level of your heads, elbows to your sides and then down to where you started.

3. Continue in sets of tens and when you get comfortable with the exercise, increase the number of times you do this routine in one set and increase the number of sets gradually.

Alternating Calf Raise

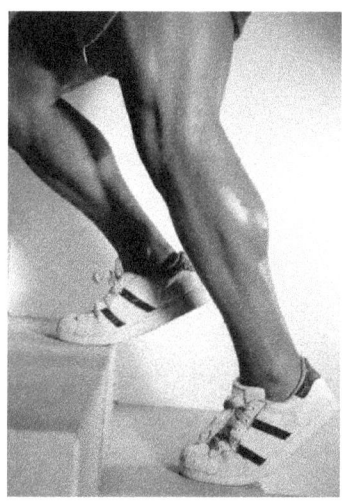

This exercise is ideal for the calves and in working your calves, this exercise also works on your stomach and helps you achieve the flat belly you have been craving for.

Here is how you will do it:

1. For this exercise, you will have to stand on a step. Keep your heels on the edge of the step and hold onto a wall for balance.

2. Continue this exercise by switching steps, lowering each towards the ground alternately.

3. To increase the intensity of the exercise and give yourself a little challenge, hold a 5-pound dumbbell in your hands and continue the exercise.

Alternating Left Hip Bridge

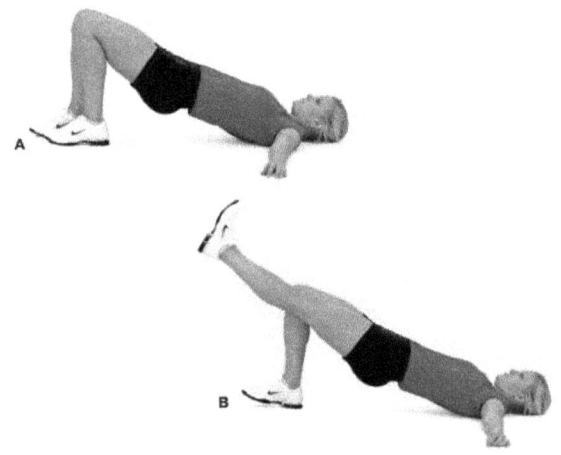

A great exercise if you are looking to build your glutes and your abs. No stability balls or dumbbells required for this one. Perform this exercise simply lying down and get results in less than two weeks.

Here is how you will do it:

1. Take your position by lying on your back. Bend your knees. Keep your hands on either side on the floor. Make sure you keep your hands flat.

2. Lift your hips up from the floor such that they are in line with your shoulders.

3. Stay in that position and straighten your left leg. Redo the same steps again in sets of ten. Switch legs with each set.

The Classic Crunch with a Twist

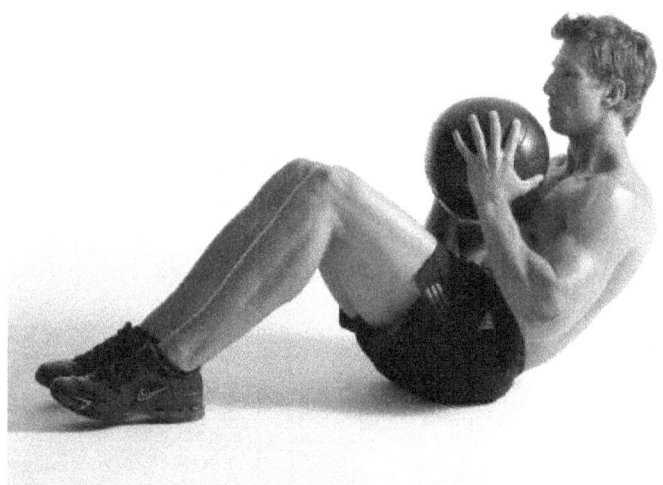

The classic crunch with a twist is an amazing exercise that will help you get rid of that muffin top in no time. Using the traditional classic crunch trick, this one uses a medicine ball to enhance the effects of the exercise.

Here is how you will do it:

1. Hold a five-pound ball in your hands, keeping your feet above the ground, swivel left and right alternately. Continue with this movement, maintaining the V shapes position.

2. It is recommended that you do this exercise two to three times a week. Start with one set and then build up to three sets in one week for best results.

Opposite Arm-Leg Reach

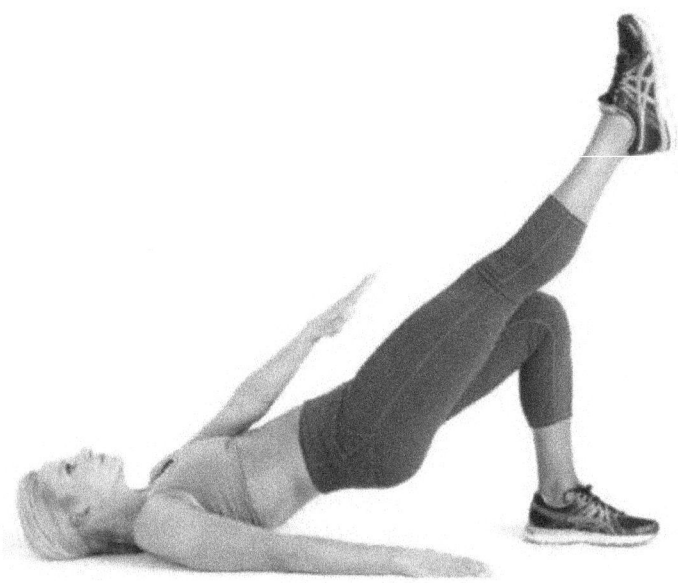

This one is another classic exercise, best for the development of lower abs. You can easily reduce your inches with this exercise while staying in one place.

Here is how you will do it:

1. Lie down on the floor with your face up and your left knee bent. Keep your left foot on the floor while your right foot should be extended towards the ceiling.

2. Keeping your right arm down to the side, use your left arm and reach your left leg with your right arm.

3. Change hands and alternately perform these steps. Continue doing this exercise in sets of 2. Ideally, do ten to twelve reps at a time.

Low Belly Leg Reach

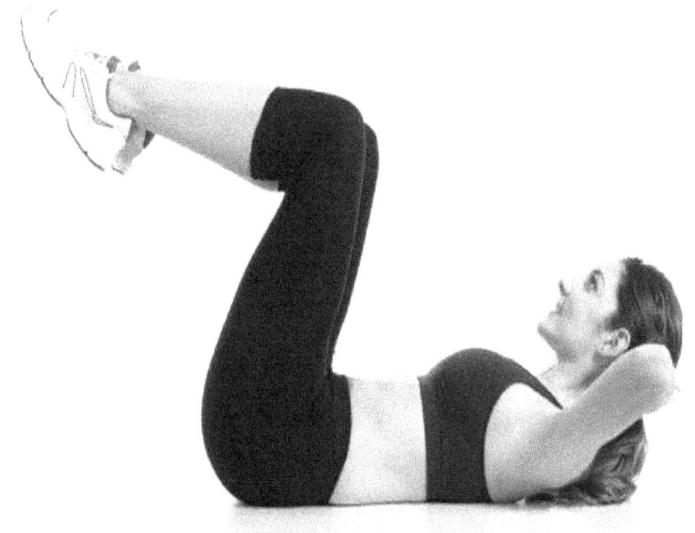

An excellent exercise to work wonders on your lower belly. Your lower abs are the hardest part to train, but this exercise makes it all very easy. Performed in one place, without any dumbbells and balls, you can do this one anywhere.

Here is how you will do it:

1. Lie down straight on the floor, facing the ceiling. Keep your knees bent at an angle of ninety degrees to the ground. Make sure your hands are on your back and your abs are contracted for best results.

2. Keep your knees over your hips, lift your shoulders up and crunch. Ideally, inhale and hold your breath for around 5 seconds.

3. Exhale and then move your legs to 45 degrees, then hold your breath again, making sure you squeeze your belly. For best results, do two sets of around 10 reps each.

Teaser

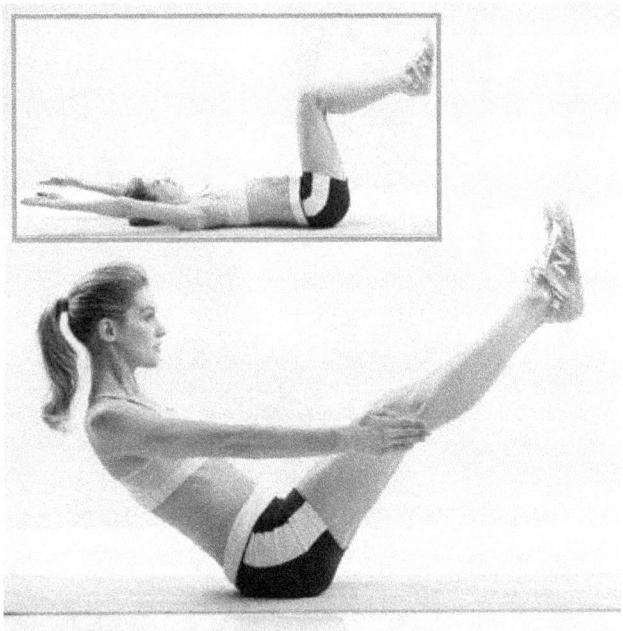

An advanced version of the classic Pilates' move that can be performed anywhere at any time just lying down. This one is great for developing your lower abs.

Here is how you will do it:

1. Lie down with your face facing the ceiling. Bend your knees at an angle of 90 degrees to your body. Keep your feet lifted.

2. Inhale to tighten your abs and then stretch your legs over your shoulder.

3. Exhale and then move your arms back to the starting position, changing the angle of your knees to 45 degrees as you move your arms. Repeat the exercise in sets of two, with ten reps in each set.

Donkey Kickbacks

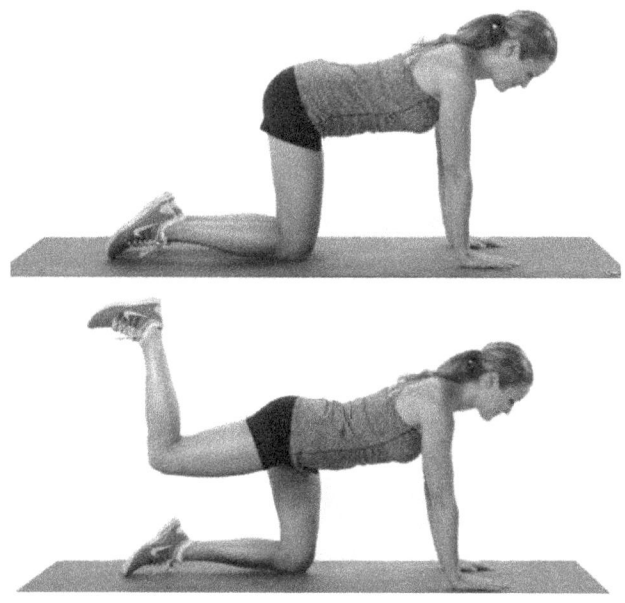

Donkey kickback is another ab exercise that will work on your entire belly and you will lose your muffin top in two weeks. This one also involves extensive movement of the legs which makes it very good for the toning of the legs.

Here is how you will do it:

1. To perform this exercise, you will first need to kneel on your knees and your arms, don't stain your back too much in this position.

2. Lift your knees two inches above the ground as you inhale and contract your abs simultaneously.

3. Next, bring your right knee to the nose, then kick your right leg straight, behind your back. Make sure you stretch your legs as far as you can. Repeat and burn calories.

Advanced Leg Crunch

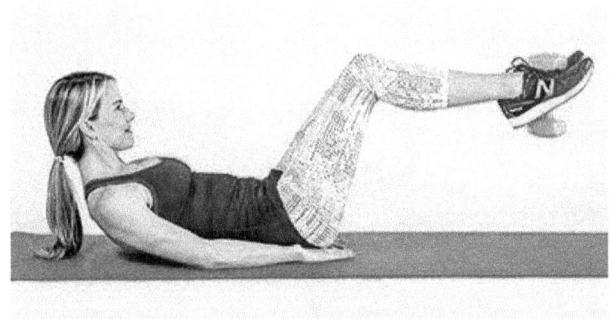

This advanced leg crunch helps you lose your calories fast. Performed easily while sitting down; this exercise only will require a place for you to lie down and you can get down to losing that belly fat.

Here is how you will do it:

1. To get started, lie on your back with your face towards the ceiling. Bend your knees, holding a three-pound dumbbell in

between them. Place your hands flat on the ground underneath your sitting bones.

2. Bring your knees towards your chest. Bring them as close as you can. Then move back to the starting position. Continue to perform in sets of ten to twenty-five.

The Belly Blaster

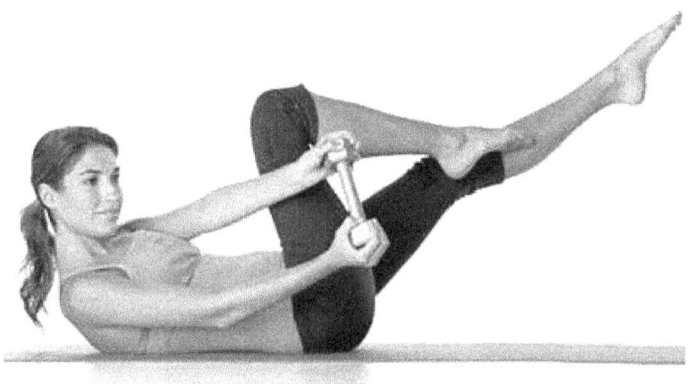

The belly blaster is great for your abs. This one is especially useful if you are looking to make six packs, this exercise is ideal for you. It will specially work on your lower abs, helping you lose your stomach in less than two weeks.

Here is how you will do it:

1. Lie on your back. Keep your knees above your chest.

2. Holding dumbbells in your hands, lifting your head and shoulders move the dumbbells from left to right, bending each knee each time. Repeat in sets.

Driving Knee Crunch

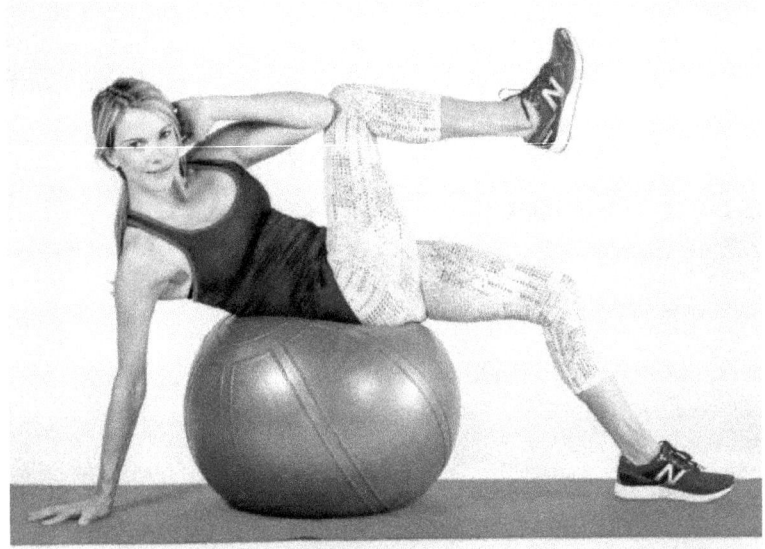

Performed with a stability ball, this one is another great ab exercise.

Here is how you will do it:

1. Lie on the stability ball with your face facing the ceiling and feet on the floor.

2. Keep your left hand on the floor for balance and with your right hand behind your head and crunch on the opposite side. Repeat in sets of two.

Scale Pose

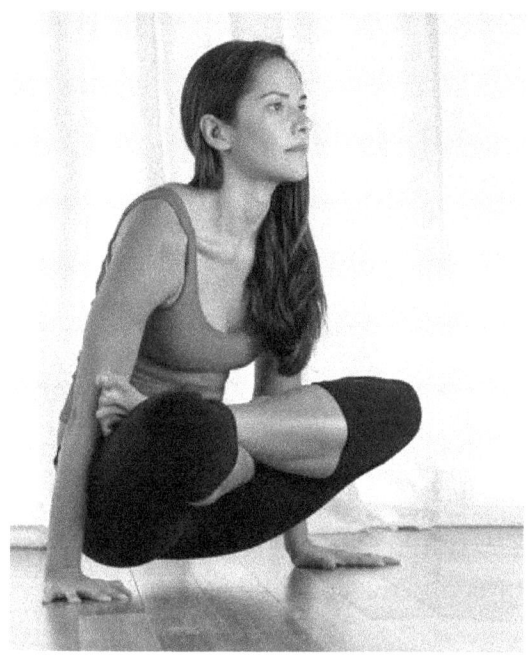

The scale pose is easy and is performed while sitting down, hands on the ground.

Here is how you will do it:

1. Sit down on a solid surface with your hands under your sitting bone.

2. Lift yourself off the ground with your hands. Repeat in sets.

The Boat Pose

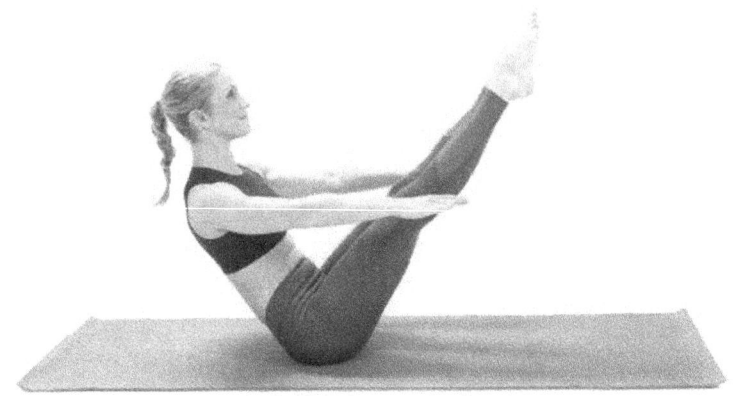

Another classic variation to the regular crunches, the boat pose works on the lower and the upper torso.

Here is how you will do it:

1. Sit down with your hands stretched out above the floor at the same angle as your legs such that you are sitting on your sitting bones.

2. Try balancing at this position, holding your breadth and then repeat.

The Cross Leg Diagonal Crunch

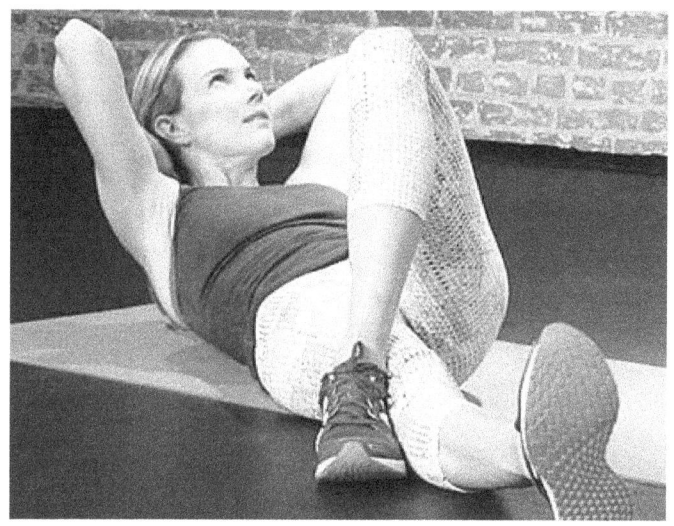

A different variation to the traditional crunch this exercise will work on your whole body, specially your torso.

Here is how you will do it:

1. Lie down on your back with your hands behind your head. Take a deep breath and straining your lower abs move your legs straight above the ground.

2. Perform the crunch by alternately taking one leg and crossing it over the other.

Tone It V-Hold

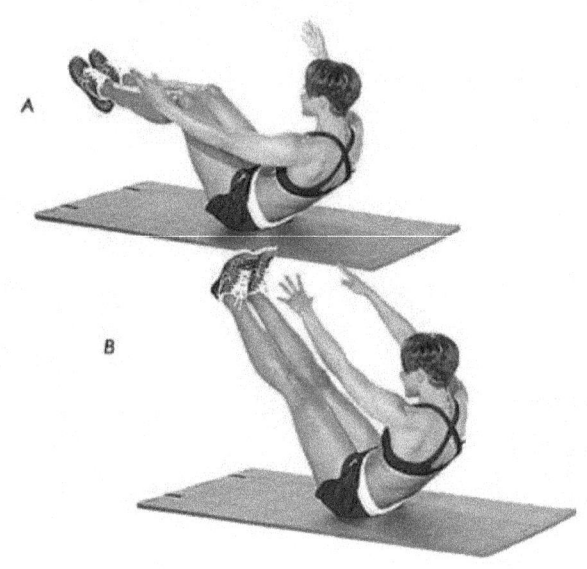

This V-hold will tone your abs like no other exercise. It gives instant results.

Here is how you will do it:

1. Lie back on your back in a V shaped position, such that your upper body and your lower body are above the ground. Try to keep your legs straight.

2. Hold your breath for as long as you can and then lie back down. Repeat.

The Plank

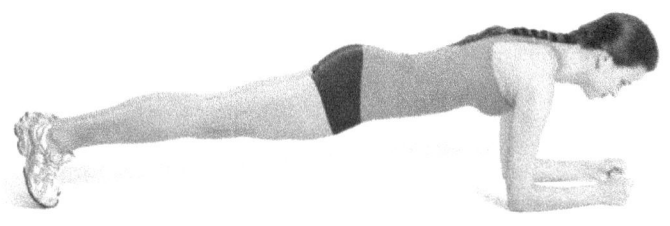

The plank will help strengthen your entire core.

Here is how you will do it:

1. Hold your body in a push up position, but with your hands stretched straight.

2. Hold your breath and hold your position for a few seconds then relax on all fours. Repeat.

Body Weight Squat

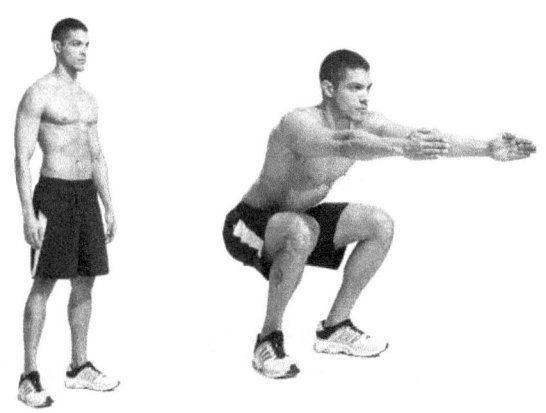

Performed while standing up, this one is easy and effective.

Here is how you will do it:

1. Standing up, with your legs shoulder-length apart, cross your arms over your chest. Squat away!

The Swan Dive

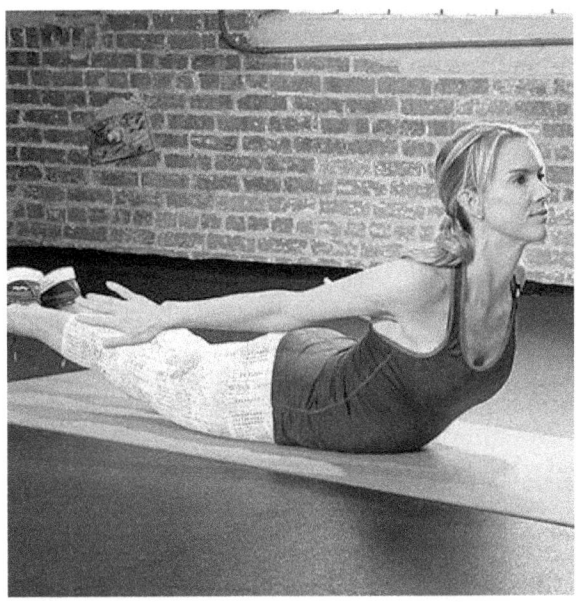

The swan dive is a modern variation to the traditional ab exercises. They are easy and effective.

Here is how you will do it:

1. Lie flat on your belly. Balance your weight while stretching your upper and lower body above the ground.

2. Hold your breath and your pose. Repeat.

Windshield Wipers

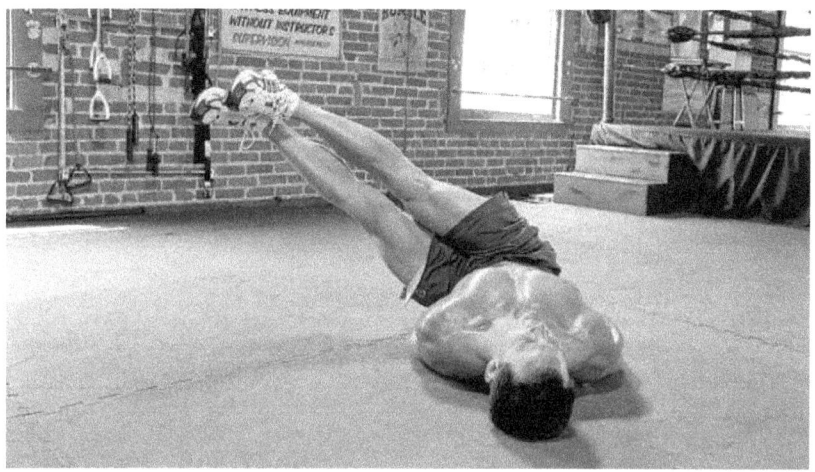

Perform this ab exercise easily while lying down. This exercise does not need any dumbbells or stability balls.

Here is how you will do it:

1. Lie flat on your back and push your knees up so they are 90 degrees from the ground. Your feet should be parallel to the ground at this position and your arms resting on the ground on either side.

2. Inhaling, move your knees to the right and back and then to your left in a windshield wiper inspired movement.

Plank on the Ball

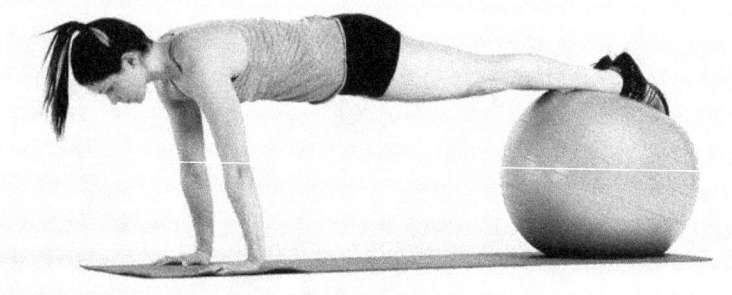

The classic plank pose is performed with a stability ball in this ab exercise.

Here is how you will do it:

1. Kneel over the stability ball with your lower body resting on the ball, feet in the air, off the ball. Rest your hands straight on the ground.

2. Hold for 30 seconds then relax. Repeat.

Jumping Jack Reach

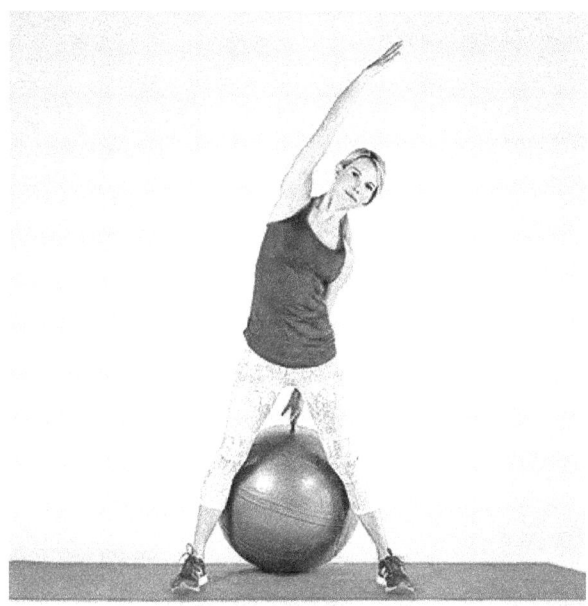

This ab exercise will take you by surprise with its results. Performed while standing up, Jumping Jack Reach will work on the entire body, tightening your muscles all over.

Here is how you will do it:

1. While sitting on the ball, jump your legs apart and then back together.

2. Next, stand you and reach left hand to your right. Repeat.

Standing Side Crunch

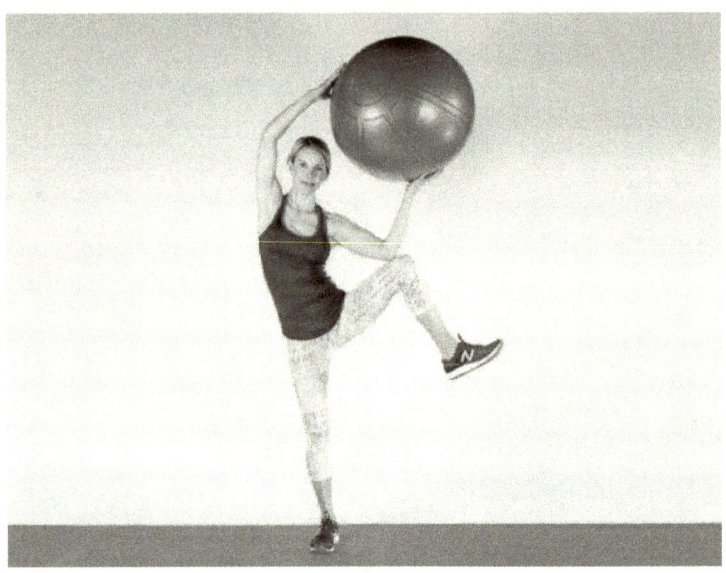

Performed while holding the stability ball in your hands, this crunch is result oriented.

Here is how you will do it:

1. Stand tall and hold the ball above your head. Keep your feet shoulder-length apart.

2. Push your right knee up to meet your elbows halfway. Repeat on the other side. Go ahead, complete the set.

The Basic Pump for Abs

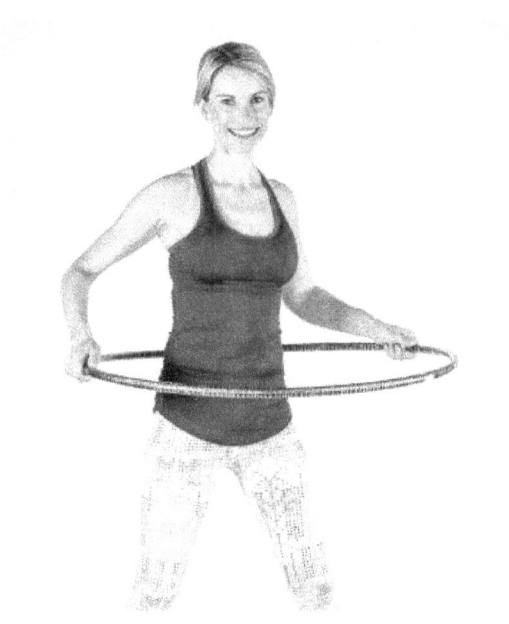

This basic pump for abs uses a hoop to achieve the perfect torso.

Here is how you will do it:

1. Stand tall with your knees slightly apart and bent.

2. Push the hoop by moving your torso around in one direction. Repeat in the other direction. Complete the set.

Circles in the Sky

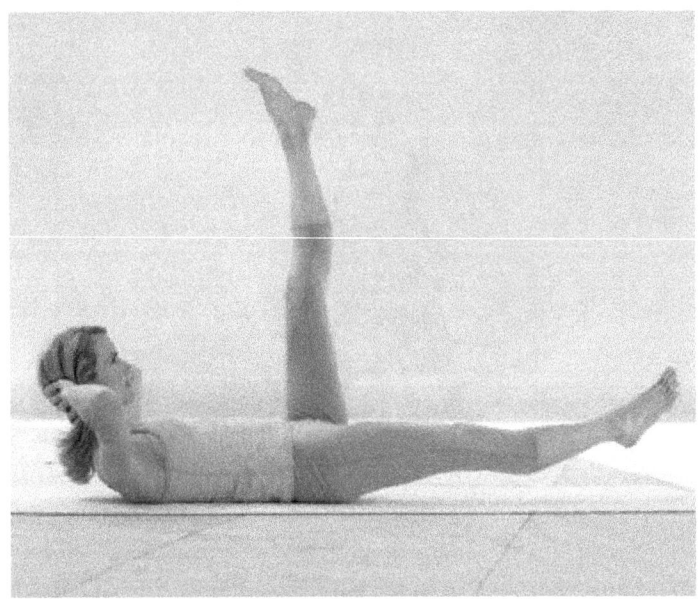

The circles in the sky are best for the core, inner thighs, the outer thigh and the butt.

Here is how you will do it:

1. Lie down facing the ceiling with your hands behind your head. Raise your upper body above the ground and one leg slightly above the ground.

2. Go all the way up with the other leg, with the leg stretched out straight at 90 degrees to the ground. Repeat the exercise with the other leg.

Side Incline with a Twist

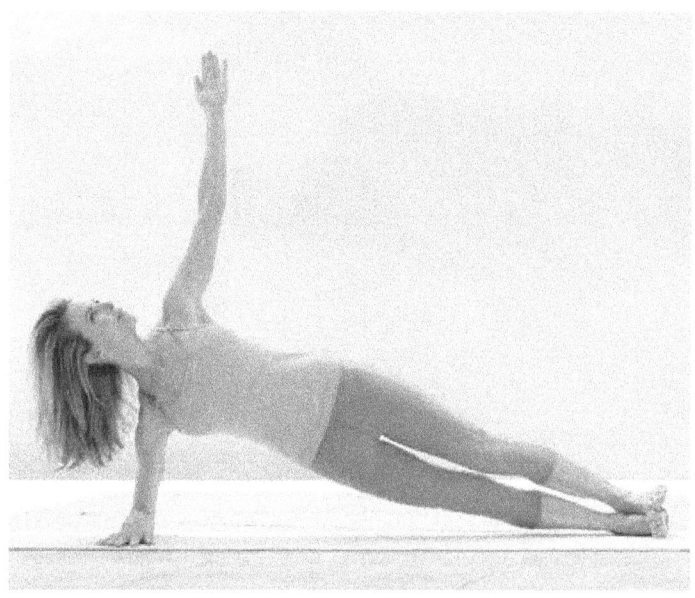

The side incline with a twist works wonders on the thighs and the core, especially the abs.

Here is how you will do it:

1. Lie on your sides with your arms perpendicular to the body. Rest your elbows on the ground for balance.

2. Using this position, try to scoop the hand extended in the air from the front of your body, through the space in between the ground and your body. Repeat.

Supine Twist

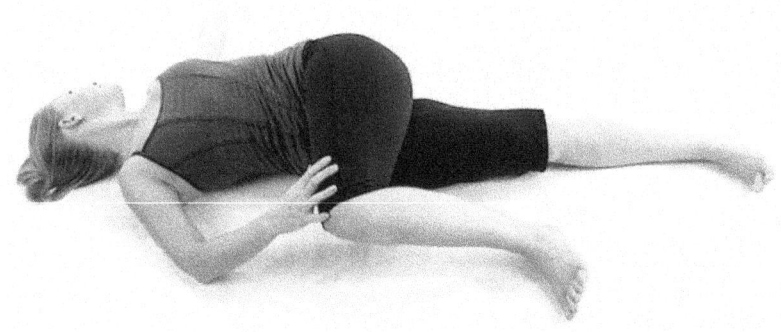

The supine twist works very well for your abs and your entire core. A variation to the traditional twist, this one is designed to help you lose more calories in less time while defining your abs.

Here is how you will do it:

1. To perform this crunch, lie straight on your back with your hands resting on either side; position your legs straight on the ground as well.

2. Now, inhale and then bring your right knee over your left as close to your chest as possible. Hug it with both your hands.

3. Use your left hand to hold the twisted knee as close to the ground as possible, stretch your right arms straight up on its side. Stretch as much as you can. Repeat on the other side.

Arms High Partial Sit-up

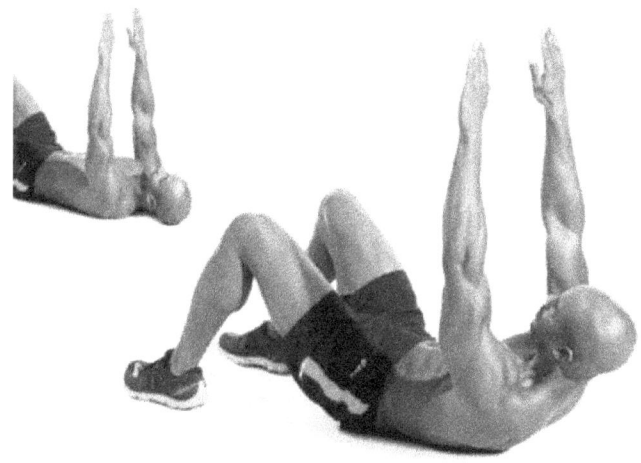

The arms high partial sit-up is designed to work efficiently on your lower abs and chest.

Here is how you will do it:

1. Lie down on your back with your knees above the ground.

2. Raise your hands straight above the ground while stretching your upper body above the ground simultaneously. Repeat.

Barbell Rollout

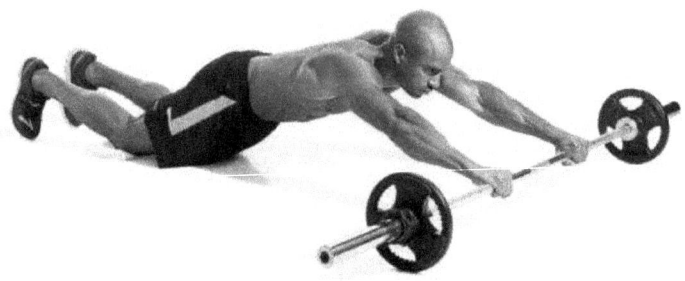

The barbell rollout helps and tones the entire body.

Here is how you will do it:

1. Kneel on the floor behind the barbell. Make sure at the start your shoulders are above the barbell.

2. Next roll the bar forward and roll forward with it, trying to keep your lower body in the same position. Roll back up and repeat.

Swiss Ball Crunch

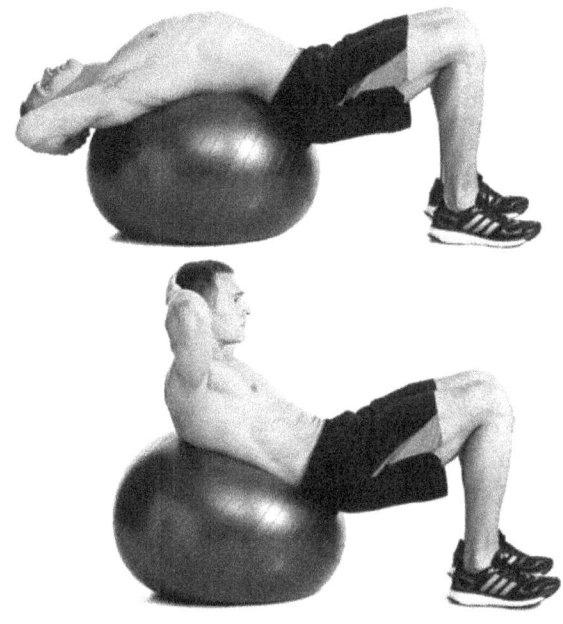

This new variation of the classic crunch is designed to add variety and faster results.

Here is how you will do it:

1. To perform this exercise, lie on the ball, with your feet on the ground, facing the ceiling. Keep your hands behind your head. In this position, you lower back is on the ball.

2. Push yourself up so that you are in a sitting position. Repeat.

Dip and Leg Raise Combo

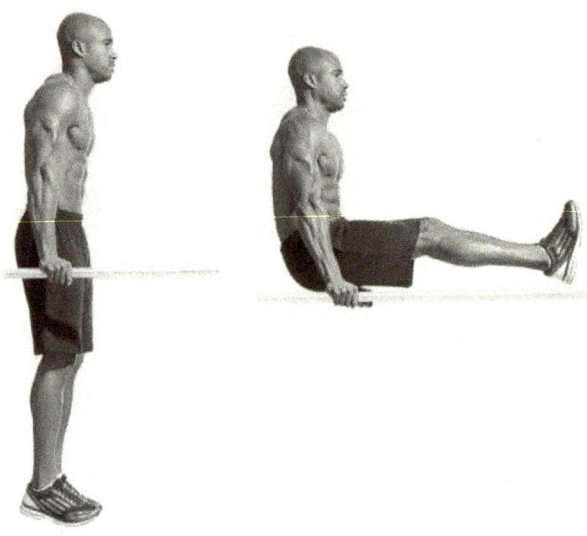

The combo is performed while suspending the air on parallel bars.

Here is how you will do it:

1. Use parallel bars and suspend yourself from the ground.

2. Bend your knees and stretch your legs right in front of you, keeping them as straight as possible. Ideally, your legs should be parallel to the ground. Repeat in sets.

Flutter Kick

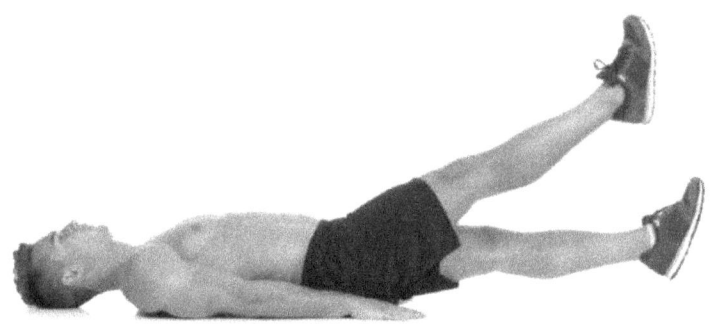

The flutter kick is easy and effective. This one does not use any bars or balls or dumbbells. The flutter kick is especially designed to improve the lower abs.

Here is how you will do it:

1. This exercise is performed by lying straight on the floor with the face facing the ceiling.

2. Force your upper and lower body slightly above the ground. Inhale at this point to increase the impact on your torso.

3. When in this position, try raising one leg slightly above the other and then back without bending them. Do the same with the other leg. Repeat in sets of two and do this exercise at least twice in one week.

Don't forget to share your thoughts on this book by leaving a review on Amazon.com. It takes just a few seconds.

Top Tips for Success

You now have all the information you need to plan a workout schedule and start making changes to your diet.

So, in this chapter, we'll focus on skincare and other things that can help you put the finishing touches on your soon-to-be toned back, butt, and legs.

Body Grooming Tips

- **Avoid Chemicals**: go for all natural or homemade lotions, moisturizers, make up, and other skin care products. The harsh chemicals found in most products can end up contributing to blemishes, wrinkles, and dry skin in the long run.

  Use products with short ingredient lists (with ingredients you can immediately identify).

  Alternatively, you can find easy recipes online to make your own products at home. This option is not only better for you and your skin, but it's also cheaper.

- **Moisturize Daily**: Use pure vegetable-based oils to deeply moisturize your skin every night before bed. Coconut oil is one of the best for this but you can also use almond oil or even olive oil.

  These are completely safe for the skin and despite being oily, will not cause blemishes. You can even use these oils as a makeup remover or moisturizer on your face. Just use a cloth to wipe away any excess so that it doesn't feel slippery.

- **Treat Yourself Weekly**: Schedule yourself regular "spa" days. This can be on your rest days from your workout. Give yourself a natural face mask (from clay or another natural material).

    Take a long bath with essential oils. Give yourself a manicure and pedicure. Just relax and pamper yourself. Even if your schedule doesn't allow you to dedicate an entire day, at least make time 1 or 2 evenings a week to spoil yourself this way.

    The treatments will improve your skin and the relaxation will help lower your stress levels (which also contributes to a younger, fresher appearance).

- **Do Weekly Hair Treatments**: During your "spa" day (or "spa" evening), include a hair treatment. Use olive oil, egg, and scented essential oils.

    Blend it into your hair until it is thoroughly coated. Pay special attention to your scalp. Leave it for 20 to 30 minutes and then rinse. This will help keep your locks strong, vibrant, and bouncy.

- **Coffee Scrubs**: Two times a week, mix coffee grounds with hot water and scrub yourself in the shower for about 10 minutes. Pay special attention to those areas with cellulite. This method has been proven to reduce cellulite and make your skin firmer and smoother. You can use the coffee grounds from the coffee you brewed that morning.

- **Lemon & Cayenne Pepper Shot**: Squeeze the juice of one lemon into a small (4 oz.) glass of water. Add 3 teaspoons of cayenne pepper. Drink.

Do this 3 times daily. You can do it with each meal, for example. Studies have shown that this can significantly reduce cellulite.

- **Use Sunscreen**: even during the winter when the sky is overcast, UV rays are still getting through. Sun damage is one of the biggest causes of premature wrinkling. Use a sunscreen with SPF no greater than 15 to protect yourself against excess sun exposure.

  Greater than 15 is not recommended as you still want to be able to absorb enough light for your body to produce vitamin D. Only use higher SPF sunscreens when you plan to spend the day lying on the beach.

- **Drink Ginger Tea**: make a tea of freshly chopped ginger, lemon juice, and a teaspoon of honey. Drink this one or two times a day.

  It's got too many health benefits to list but it also helps slow the breakdown of elastin in your skin (the protein that is responsible for keeping your skin from sagging).

Tips for Staying Motivated

- **One Day at a Time**: Rather than letting yourself get overwhelmed by the long road ahead of you, focus on improving yourself one day at a time.

  At the end of each day, write down your goals for the next day. The next day, focus specifically on those goals. It's good to have long-term goals but it's equally important to have short term goals that can help you get there.

- **Bounce Back**: if you miss a day of workout because you couldn't find the motivation, don't beat yourself up about it. Just get up the next day and get back on schedule.

- **Take a 30-Day Challenge**: commit to making these serious changes for at least 30 days. You will start to notice weight loss results quickly once you start working out and cutting down on processed foods but the most dramatic results will not start to appear until at least 30 days.

  It also takes about 3 to 4 weeks for new habits to settle in and become routine. So, before you make any major decisions about giving up or trying something else, give your current plan at least 30 days to take effect before you consider making any changes.

- **Record Your Progress**: keep a journal which contains your goals, progress, and emotions. Write in it daily so that you have a clear and detailed record of your progress. It should include things like:
    - 1 Year Goals
    - 1 Month Goals
    - 1 Week Goals
    - 1 Day Goals
    - Current waistline, current weight, etc.
    - Goal waistline, goal weight, etc.
    - Workout schedule
    - Weekly menu
    - Brief descriptions of how you feel before and after your workout
    - Brief descriptions of how you feel before and after meals

- **Reward Yourself**: positive reinforcement is more effective than negative reinforcement. Keep yourself motivated by giving yourself small rewards once per week or once per month.

  This reward could even be your "spa" day or it could be a small shopping trip to buy a hot new dress that will show off your future beautiful backside!

Discover Scientifically-Proven "Shortcuts" & "Hacks" to Lose Weight FASTER (With Very Little Effort)

For this month only, you can get Linda's best-selling & most popular book absolutely free – *Weight Loss Secrets You NEED to Know*.

Get Your FREE Copy Here:

TopFitnessAdvice.com/Bonus

Discover scientifically-proven tips to help you lose weight faster and easier than ever before. With this book, readers were able to improve their weight loss results and fitness levels. So, it's highly recommended that you get this book, especially while it's free!

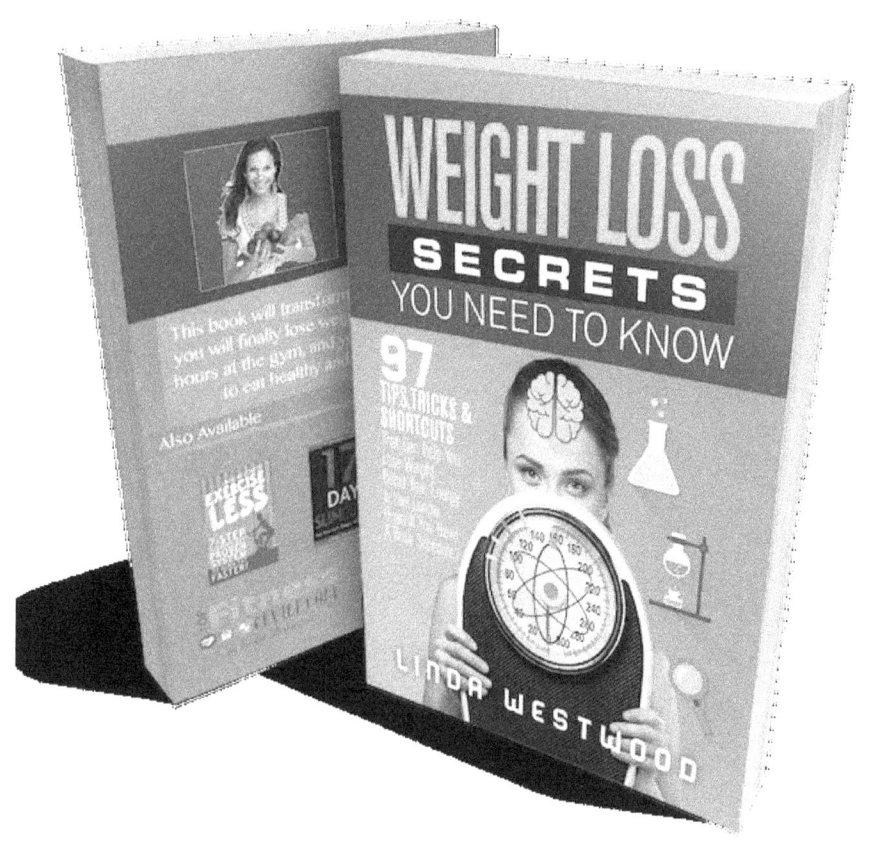

Get Your FREE Copy Here:
TopFitnessAdvice.com/Bonus

Conclusion

Using this detailed guide, you can now create weekly workout and meal plans that will help you build muscle, lose weight, and achieve that perfect, shapely body that will look hot from behind—and from the front, side, or any other angle!

Getting down to your goal figure takes motivation and commitment. But more importantly: it takes good planning. If you want to achieve that perfect body and stay there; don't treat diet and exercise like a sprint.

Treat them like a marathon. That means, don't rush at full speed as soon as the shot is fired. Start at a steady pace that won't tire you out right at the beginning.

Start by working out 3 times a week for 15 minutes (plus an extra 20 for the warm up and cool down). After the first week, you can increase it to 4 times a week. Then, do 5 times a week.

Always give yourself 1 day of rest for every 3 days that you work out. Your body needs some time to focus on repairing the tears in your muscles and building them up so that they will be ready to take on more the next time. This will end up being 1-2 rest days per week.

Once you start to feel yourself getting used to a certain exercise, bump up the intensity to keep it challenging. If you keep it at the same intensity all the time, your body will hit a plateau and stop growing new muscles.

When it comes to transitioning to a healthy diet, take a positive approach. Don't think of it as a "diet" that you will do just until the weight is gone.

This is a lifestyle change. That said, if you cut out *all* the foods you are used to eating at once, you are going to probably experience withdrawal systems like intense cravings. Instead, swap out foods on a weekly basis.

Each Sunday, choose 3 unhealthy foods that you eat regularly and eliminate these from your diet for that week. At the same time that you pick 3 unhealthy foods to eliminate, choose 3 healthy foods that you can eat instead. The next Sunday, choose another 3 unhealthy foods to replace with 3 healthy foods.

That week, you are allowed to eat the 3 unhealthy foods that you eliminated the week before.

The goal is not to make your diet boring and totally uninteresting. A candy bar or ho-ho every now and again are not going to ruin all your hard work.

The goal of this transition is to break your habit of eating too much junk food and getting your body used to eating primarily healthy food.

Giving up 3 unhealthy foods for a week and then reintroducing them (while you eliminate another 3 unhealthy foods) will make the transition easier because you know that all you have to do is make it through 1 week without those foods.

At the same time, it will give you the chance to realize that you *can* go a whole week without eating 3 of the foods you once ate on a daily basis. The week that you reintroduce those foods, it will be easier to moderate your consumption of them. Just because you reintroduce them doesn't mean you should start eating or drinking them daily again.

Instead, all yourself just 1 or 2 portions during the week as a special treat.

Your tastes will begin to change as you learn to taste other flavors aside from salt and sugar. It might not seem possible now but processed foods will soon start to taste awful to you. The main ingredients in these foods are either artificial or just a lot of salt and sugar.

These are the 2 most basic flavors that our body craves but there is a world of different flavors out there that you can only appreciate when they aren't being masked over by excessive salt and sugar. As you start to introduce more whole, healthy foods, you'll start to appreciate and crave these flavors.

Take it one day at a time and don't let yourself be discouraged by mistakes and setbacks.

These things might feel like you have taken a step backwards but they are actually a sign that you are moving forward.

Mistakes and setbacks mean that you are actually challenging yourself and your body to do better. Embrace them and learn from them.

Use this book as a reference guide and a source of inspiration as you embark on your own journey to slim down and finally get that perfect back, butt, and legs you have always dreamed of!

Enjoying this book?

Check out my other best sellers!

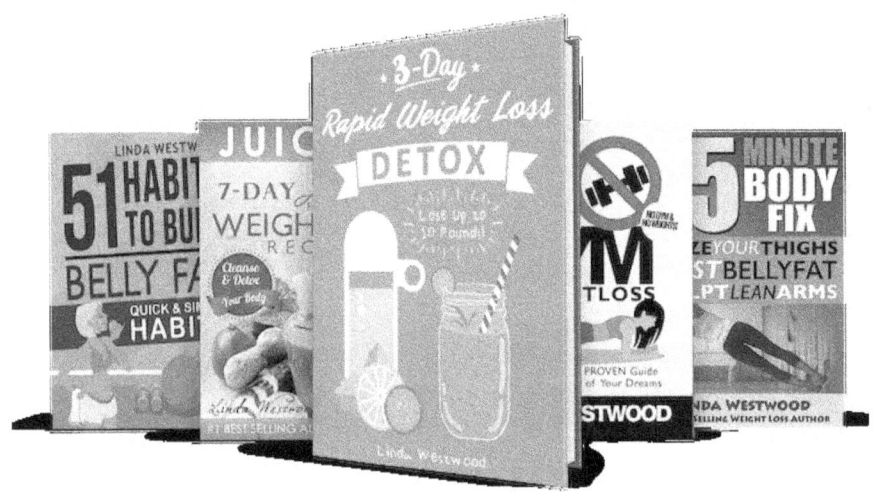

Get your next book on sale here:

TopFitnessAdvice.com/go/books

Final Words

I would like to thank you for purchasing my book and I hope I have been able to help you and educate you on something new.

If you have enjoyed this book and would like to share your positive thoughts, could you please take 30 seconds of your time to go back and give me a review on my Amazon book page.

I greatly appreciate seeing these reviews because it helps me share my hard work.

You can leave me a review on Amazon.com.

Again, thank you and I wish you all the best!

www.ingramcontent.com/pod-product-compliance
Lightning Source LLC
Chambersburg PA
CBHW031144020426
42333CB00013B/506